The Fat Fix Diet

Using Homeopathic HCG

The Fat Fix Diet
Using Homeopathic HCG

The Natural Solution to Unnatural Fat

Anne Dunev, Ph.D.

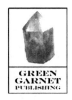

GREEN
GARNET
PUBLISHING

Disclaimer

The contents of this book are not meant to be used as a medical diagnosis, nor for the treatment of any disease. Before making any dietary changes, please consult your physician or health care practitioner.

Contents

Plateau
49

Acknowledgements

Writing a book is a Labor of Love. The writing part is Love and all that comes after is Labor! It takes quite a few people in the Delivery Room to help bring forth the finished product.

So, I want to thank Alan Gilbertson for his editing, design and sage advice, Deanna Noll for her proof-reading, my son Nick Dunev for his editing and cover design, my son Lucas Dunev for his photography and making his mom look good and Michael Duff for helping me look better through his photo shop skills. My husband Peter helped with editing and was resident cheerleader.

Everyone at the office where I practice, Lisa Benest, MD in Burbank, CA, has been very helpful to me. The staff is terrific and some were the first to volunteer for the FAT FIX DIET. Their feedback and ultimate successes launched the program. You can find photos of our staff at www.lisabenestmd.com

I want to thank all the patients and friends who have done the FAT FIX DIET and gave me their suggestions, success stories, recipes and enthusiasm for this program. I learned so much from them. Also, thanks to my Distributors who gave me the benefit of their experiences. It has been a pleasure to hear how the Distributors are helping others achieve their weight loss and health goals.

My adventure in Nutrition began at age 4 when I used to watch Jack La Lanne with my babysitter and she made me sandwiches from Jack's whole grain protein bread. Jack passed away today at the age of 96. I owe him for my very first exposure to "health food". I told my Mom that I didn't want the white bread served at our house, but I liked the taste of the Jack La Lanne bread. Jack was a great inspiration to so many people and I wish him bon voyage on his journey to his next adventure.

Adelle Davis was my next influence. I found her books in college, just when I was studying Health Sciences at Ohio State University. Adelle taught me that food could be medicine and that there were solutions in nutrients and a Nature-based approach that could never be found in pharmaceuticals. From there the list is long, and distinguished: Dr. Royal Lee, Dr. Weston Price, Dr. Melvin Page, Dr. Francis Pottenger, to name a few.

I am very fortunate to have found good friends and wise teachers, and I am grateful to all of them. With this book I hope that my good fortune is passed on to others.

Preface

What is "unnatural" fat? Ask yourself—is there any fat on your body that you feel does not belong there? Do you have fat in places where you did not have fat when you were younger, or fitter or slimmer?

Each person usually knows for his or her own body which fat is unnatural. There is a basic shape to the human body that follows a standard blueprint. With the current obesity epidemic we are seeing wild variations in that shape. Bloating, inflammation and water retention give bodies distorted shapes.

The FAT FIX DIET eating plan, along with Homeopathic HCG, will help you lose weight where you need to lose it most. Bloat and inflammation will be reduced. You can reshape your body without spending all your time at the gym or starving yourself, or taking dangerous drugs.

The road to healthy eating is also the road to a shapely body. This means that you will feel better, have more energy and enjoy life more, while you are losing weight faster than ever before.

Anne Dunev
Los Angeles

Welcome to the Fat Fix Diet Program

Thanks for your interest in the FAT FIX DIET Program. This is a tool that you can use to help make your life easier. Whether you want to lose 10 pounds or 100 pounds, there is a safe and effective boost to speed you on your way.

The FAT FIX DIET is simple to follow. It may not be easy at times, because the vast majority of us have habits to break, and that can be a challenge. But the rewards will be worth it! Patients and friends contact me every day to thank me for introducing them to this diet plan.

I want to thank Dr. A.T.W. Simeons who started it all when he developed the prescription version of the HCG diet. There are many doctors who have taught me about hormones, blood sugar and nutrition. All that I have learned in many years of study and practice is incorporated into my own version of the HCG diet, using homeopathic HCG to create the FAT FIX DIET Program.

In this manual you will find the original protocol from Dr. Simeons, a 500 calorie diet, and you are welcome to follow that program. You will also find my version, which is about 800–1000 calories. When it comes to blood sugar balance, it is not calories that are important, but maintaining consistent blood sugar so that the body does not constantly store new fat. This also seems

[handwritten notes in right margin: "illegal?" / "See Mayo site" / "+ dangerous" / "Used for fertility —"]

to allow the HCG to work so that fat loss is accelerated, and the metabolism reset, just as Dr. Simeons discovered.

Many patients seem to lose as much weight on my program as patients who follow Dr. Simeons' diet and use prescription injections of actual HCG hormones. Some who have done both my Homeopathic HCG version and Dr. Simeons' say that the prescription HCG hormone is a bit stronger in terms of appetite control. Others report they see no difference in the amount of weight lost or diminished appetite. People still lose weight and excess fat deposits on all versions of HCG. Dr. Simeons recommended that 26 pounds is the maximum amount of weight that should be lost in 40 days. Many of my patients have achieved that goal using the homeopathic HCG version along with the FAT FIX DIET plan. Just as Dr. Simeons described, their bodies are also reshaped on the homeopathic version. Fat is lost where they want to lose it, and their metabolism is reset so they seem to burn their food more efficiently afterwards and not regain weight as easily as they did before.

Like most things in life, you will get out of the FAT FIX DIET what you put in. The patients who strictly follow the program lose better. This manual tries to cover all the possible questions that come up, and any glitches in rapid loss so that anyone can achieve their weight goals.

How Can You Stick To A Diet?

It is easy to lose weight. Feed someone only bread and water for 6 months and they will lose weight. Or feed just rice and vegetables, or anything that provides a small amount of calories, but keeps a body alive.

So, there is little problem with losing weight. But losing weight may also involve losing health, and that's a problem. Bread and water alone will cause many nutritional deficiencies, and subsequent health problems. If you have any doubts about the value of nutrition check out the photos of people who have been prisoners of war or survived concentration camps.

Let's look at the difference between nutrition and food. Nutrition is essential vitamins, minerals, fats and proteins needed by cells for fuel, repair and creation of functioning new cells. Food is anything we put in our mouths and swallow.

Rice and vegetables might be slightly better, especially if the rice is whole brown rice. But both of these diets lack essential nutrients and will lead to severe health issues and disease states.

Deprivation of food is not the problem for most of us. Deprivation of essential nutrients is a problem for most of us, no matter how much food we are consuming. It is the abundance of food and the constant temptation that makes it hard to stick to a diet long enough to lose weight. And it is the abundance of food that tastes good, offers comfort or release from cares and worries, but gives little or no nourishment to the cells of the body, that is making us fat—and sick.

When Dieting is Not Enough

Some people do try to starve themselves—and still the weight does not come off. They may be accused of closet eating. But the problem is not always how much they are eating; it is what the body is doing with the food inside the body. It is not as simple as calories consumed and calories burned, especially as the body ages, or if there is hormonal imbalance.

Hormones play a very large factor in body fat and in the distribution of body fat. This should come as no surprise. Hormones cause breasts to develop, voices to get deep and muscles build. Hormones have everything to do with the size and shape of our bodies. Ask any woman who has been through puberty, pregnancy and menopause how much difference hormones make in the shape of her body!

Many people feel out of control of their weight, but it is possible to get back some control, through safe and effective nutritional supplements, and a correct eating plan that helps balance the hormones that determine fat storage and distribution.

I am convinced, after many years of helping people improve their health through natural means, that you cannot be healthy relying on Western medicine and pharmaceutical drugs, which are synthetic chemicals. We have been led to believe that only drugs can make us well. In some cases, pharmaceuticals can be life-saving. But the basic constitution and health of the body is determined by the health and integrity of the cells. The only way to build and repair cells is by supplying cellular building blocks through nutrition. What Nature puts into food is what our cells need.

The modern chronic diseases of heart disease, diabetes, cancer and obesity are caused mostly by eating the wrong types of food or eating chemical, factory made and processed foods.

The Fastest, Easiest, Healthiest Diet in the World

Hundreds of people have lost weight with the FAT FIX DIET plan. Although the homeopathic HCG seems like "magic" it is the combination of the eating plan, plus the homeopathic

HCG drops, which jump-starts your loss so that you will lose faster than ever before.

The FAT FIX DIET program is safe because it is based on sound health principles. The diet will balance your blood sugar, which has great health benefits beyond weight loss.

This is not "hormone replacement," but it appears to tweak your system to accelerate fat burning. Homeopathic medicine has been around since the 1700s and is widely used in Europe. There have been no problems reported with the Homeopathic HCG and it is safe to use with prescription medications. Of course, please consult your health practitioner and/or medical doctor if you are on a medical program before starting any weight loss regimen.

You do not need to count calories on the Fat Fix plan. Simply eat according to the instructions, confining your food choices to proteins, fruits and vegetables, with 2 bread sticks, Melba toasts or crackers allowed per day.

I have used diets that balance blood sugar to help people lose weight for many years and it does work. The reason that you add the Homeopathic HCG is because it accelerates your weight loss so that you will lose pounds from the first few days. Many people will lose a pound per day, but not everyone. Men tend to lose faster than women. Obese people lose faster than merely over-weight people. *Everyone can lose weight on the Fat Fix plan* if they do the diet, and follow the instructions in this book. There are lots of tips to follow, and questionnaires to answer, so that you can understand much more about your individual metabolism and what your body needs to stay slim and healthy.

Another reason to use the Homeopathic HCG is because it causes the body to drop inches better than anything I have ever seen. It is common to lose 1-2 dress sizes or belt sizes in one round of the FAT FIX DIET Plan. One round is 4-6 weeks.

Obese or just slightly over-weight people can use this diet plan. It is healthy for anyone. You will be able to maintain the weight loss if you do the Maintenance strictly and follow the Forever After advice.

There are only a few things you need to do to get started. Many people find this is the easiest, quickest most enjoyable diet they have ever done. Your life may never be the same again.

The Secret of HCG

HCG is a secret weapon to help balance your hormones and help you stick to a diet. Containing no drugs or herbs that suppress appetite, HCG helps you to eat less the same way your body does. After a big meal, there is sufficient sugar and fat circulating in your blood for the body to get the signal to stop eating.

No one who has lost weight using Homeopathic HCG doubts that this program is very effective, and that the weight loss is faster, easier and more targeted than any other weight loss program they have tried before.

The HCG drops appear to trigger the slow release of fat from the stored fat in your own extra padding in the belly, waist, hips, thighs and rear. The intelligence of the body does not allow release of fat from places where it is needed to cushion, protect or contour. For example, there is brown fat that helps control temperature, but does not add bulk. HCG will not mobilize this fat.

The fat that is triggered by the HCG is used by the body for fuel and repair. The extra fat released by the HCG is used for energy until your mirror tells you that you have a younger, more pleasing shape, your clothing size diminishes, and your friends start to ask what you are doing to look so good.

Don't go out of your weigh to please anyone but yourself.

Author Unknown

7

The interesting thing is that inches of weight are lost, along with the pounds, but the skin does not become slack. Have you ever seen someone over 50 who lost a large amount of weight in a short period of time? Often the hanging turkey neck from the weight loss makes them look older than the extra pounds ever did. This does not happen on the HCG diet. In every case I have seen, after the HCG program, the face and neck look firm and youthful, despite the age of the dieter. The face may look thinner and a little fat, plus a lot of bloat, may be lost. But never enough to make the skin sag.

Often the body is holding water to dilute toxins. A toxin is a substance that is destructive to cells because the body cannot break it down into non-harmful bits. Arsenic is a metal that is toxic in large quantities. Pesticides are toxins that attack the nervous system. Remember that if something is strong enough to kill bugs, it is strong enough to kill human cells also. The Nazi final solution was a nerve gas that was actually a pesticide.

Too little protein and too much sugar and starch can also cause water retention. Shift the diet to meats, fish, fruits and vegetables, and excess water is excreted.

Inflammation diminishes, also. Some people report less aches, pains, allergies and digestive difficulties.

It is very important to drink enough water. The body needs plenty of water to keep the correct salt ratio in the blood so that waste can be passed out of the cells. Drink about half your body weight in ounces of water. If you weigh 150 lbs, drink at least 75 ounces, or 9-10 glasses of filtered or spring water.

What Kind of Food is Allowed?

Because the American food supply is filled with chemicals, hormones, medications, artificial colors and flavors, many people do not know what it is like to eat real food. The diet you must follow on the Homeopathic HCG program is a diet stripped of artificial additives and takes you back to the basics of natural food.

That does not mean the food has to be tasteless or boring. Spices and condiments can be enjoyed in abundance, as long as they do not contain oils or sugar or anything artificial.

Garlic, onion, lemon juice, soy sauce, basil, chili pepper, basil, oregano, etc, will give your food a gourmet twist so that sticking to the diet becomes possible, and even enjoyable.

Many people have developed HCG friendly recipes and some of those are featured here to inspire you.

What is HCG and
How Does it Work?

HCG[1] is a hormone produced in quantity during pregnancy that may be detected in blood or urine by a pregnancy test. It is a naturally occurring protein hormone that develops in the placenta during the first trimester of pregnancy shortly after conception.

This protein hormone is recognized as a peptide. Peptides are a class of hormone that is secreted into the blood stream and aide in endocrine functions in living animals. Men and non-pregnant women also produce HCG.

HCG is believed to help reset the hypothalamus by sending signals to begin breaking down and using abnormally high body fat as a primary fuel source. These signals may be sent when the body is experiencing a reduced and low calorie diet. It is also believed that these signals send a message out to conserve and maintain lean body mass, i.e., muscle mass. Without HCG to assist you during a low calorie diet, your body will begin to deplete muscle, and you may be very hungry.

The original HCG diet program was developed by Dr. A.T.W. Simeons actual pharmaceutical HCG hormone

I bought a talking refrigerator that said "Oink" every time I opened the door. It made me hungry for pork chops.

Marie Mott

---

1   HCG is Human Chorionic Gonadotropin, with the following Latin roots: *chorion* = fetal membrane, *gonad* = ovary or testes, *trop* = to affect.

shots, injected 6 days out of 7 for 3-6 weeks. This method is by prescription and thus expensive, running hundreds to thousands of dollars, depending upon the doctor.

I have used natural homeopathic medicine for years in my practice with great success. I was interested in seeing if the homeopathic version of HCG was just as effective as the prescription version. The staff in my office volunteered to try it, and were very happy with the results. People report that they can immediately feel the difference when they use the drops, and they lose their hunger. In both the prescription HCG (injections or drops) and the Homeopathic drops, spray or pellets, the results appear to be the same.

The Magic Drops™ Homeopathic HCG drops are from an FDA certified laboratory in the U.S.A. The FDA regulates proper preparation of homeopathic medicines.

Homeopathic medicines are made by diluting active substances. The medicines trigger the immune system to correct a condition. Scientifically it can not yet be explained precisely how homeopathy works, but new theories in quantum physics are shedding light on the process. What we do know is that a carefully selected homeopathic remedy acts as a trigger to the body's healing processes. We know this because of the results that occur when homeopathy is used.

This is called "Functional Medicine." Improved function is the proof that the remedy was successful.

The homeopathic version of HCG is not hormone replacement, which makes it very safe to use, but the body responds in a similar way to the injected HCG.

Drops

Homeopathy can be used without a prescription, there are no injections, and it is easy to travel with the remedy and use it on your schedule.

The Three Different Types of HCG

HCG is a hormone produced by the hypothalamus gland. Men and non-pregnant women have small amounts, but HCG is produced in great amounts during pregnancy. The hormone ensures that the woman's body will break down fat to nourish and sustain the developing baby, if needed. For purposes of using HCG for weight loss, there are three types available.

Prescription HCG Injections. This must be prescribed by a medical doctor or is available over the internet. This is actual HCG hormone.

- Oral Prescription HCG. This may be prescribed by a medical doctor or is available over the internet. The prescription hormone is mixed and then used as drops taken by mouth.

- Homeopathic HCG. Available currently as tincture (drops) or as a spray. No prescription is necessary. Magic Drops™ recommended in the Fat Fix Diet™ Plan are Homeopathic HCG. This is an extremely dilute form of the actual HCG hormone. At a certain level of dilution, the homeopathic remedy becomes "activated".

HCG ordered over the internet from India or China arrives as a powder that must be mixed with a liquid. It is then taken orally (by mouth) and must be refrigerated. This is prescription HCG.

13

A few compounding pharmacists do make prescription HCG to be used as oral drops.

Homeopathic HCG should be manufactured in American FDA certified laboratories according to established homeopathic standards. This is a point to check wherever you purchase homeopathic HCG. Magic Drops ™ Homeopathic HCG is produced at an FDA certified lab.

There appears to be some confusion about the type of fat burned when using different types of HCG. Dr. Simeons talked about burning fat reserves, but leaving the structural fat that supports the organs. All forms of HCG burn the "right" kind of fat. The evidence of this is that all forms of HCG resculpt the body.

You will lose fat where you need to lose it, from your "fluffiest" parts. Most people get excess fat deposit in the waist when they have a metabolic imbalance, produced when there is too much insulin. That is why the sugar balancing program in the FAT FIX DIET is effective. It is also an insulin-balancing program, as is Dr. Simeons very low calorie diet. Reduce insulin levels and the body will plug into your reserve tank of fat and burn the fat for fuel to the muscles.

One of the most astonishing things about using HCG for weight loss is that the skin contracts in ratio to the loss of pounds. That means that people do not get the loose skin and turkey neck that sometimes happens with other types of reducing plans.

All forms of HCG are effective, so choose the plan that seems like the best one for you.

The Magic Drops
and Your Fat

Patients and friends call me all the time to request more of the "Magic Drops". And the HCG drops do seem magic, when you consider the past failed diets so many people have tried.

But the drops alone are not enough to reduce pounds and inches, reshape the body and reset the metabolism.

The Magic Drops only work when the internal "climate" of the body is changed with the eating plan. While you are taking the Drops, your body will let go of the fat from your own fat cells. This mobilized fat will help make up for the lack of fat in your meals.

The eating program for the FAT FIX DIET plan is very healthy. Eliminating the starches (grains and potatoes and pastas) and the sugar allows the body to stop making the fat that is now being stored in your thighs, waist and bum. And, very quickly, the body will start unlocking the extra fat cells and releasing the stored fat so that you can use it for fuel, and for the care and repair of cells.

The Phase 3 Maintenance program, which adds fat back into the diet, is an ideal way to eat long term. I advise you to consider the Maintenance program as your steady life style, with occasional deviations, and treats. If we had all eaten according to the Maintenance plan 90% of the time, probably none of us would need the HCG drops now!

Phase 2 of the FAT FIX DIET eating plan, the no-fat plan you follow while taking the Drops, is only a temporary program that I do not recommend as an everyday life style because of the lack of dietary fat. The protein, fruits and vegetables, no sugar, no grains, is fine. But avoiding all dietary fat is not a healthy way to eat, unless you are taking the HCG drops.

Fat is essential for your body. Every cell in the body has fat in the membrane of the cell. Vitamins attach to fats in order to get absorbed so they can be used. Fats such as fish oils are anti-inflammatory. Fats in raw coconut oil help to make the intestines healthy. Even the fat in meat and eggs is fat your body can use. It is not true that these fats go straight to the arteries. Only 10% of cholesterol is from dietary fat. The rest of cholesterol is made in your liver—from sugar and starches, not from fat.

Confused about fats? Scientists cannot agree about fat, either, so you are not alone. It is easy to see why fat got such a bad reputation. Eat fat and you get fat, right? Seems logical, except that it just isn't true. Cultures where a high amount of dietary fat is consumed are some of the healthiest in the world.

For example, Inuit people (Eskimos) natively ate mostly blubber and protein, but were strong, lean and almost free of degenerative diseases like cancer or heart disease. Vitamin C, which humans cannot synthesize and must obtain from dietary sources, was supplied by eating the adrenal glands of animals. B vitamins were stored in organ meats, such as the liver. When Inuits and Native Americans started eating the White Man's diet of white sugar, white flour and coffee, with little fat or protein, cancer, obesity and heart disease became rampant seemingly over-night.

In the liver the body makes cholesterol and triglycerides out of sugars and starches, candy, cake, breads and pastas. Triglycerides can be burned by the body for fuel, but excess triglycerides are converted to fat and stored—in your hips and stomach.

Cholesterol medications work by inhibiting your liver from converting sugars and starches into cholesterol. This may sound like a good idea, but messing with or inhibiting natural liver function is a very dicey proposition. The liver is the main detoxification organ in the body. Liver function must be monitored closely and many people cannot tolerate cholesterol medications. Since there is little evidence that lowering cholesterol really improves heart disease, natural dietary solutions are much safer approach. The FAT FIX DIET plan has helped many people lower their cholesterol, if you are concerned about it. Remember that the body makes sex hormones out of cholesterol, and the fat membrane that protects cells are made from fat. So, fat is not our enemy. But sugars and starches may well be. Sugars and starches are not necessary for health. Perhaps it is no accident that fat makes foods taste good.

So, when should you have started eating this way? Twenty years ago. That would have been best. Second best is starting to eat that way from the moment you finish your HCG drops.

One of the most exciting things about the FAT FIX DIET with FAT FIX DIET Homeopathic HCG is that it is never too late to reclaim your youthful shape. That has given some a brighter outlook on their future, no matter their age.

How Homeopathy Works

Many medical doctors do not understand homeopathic principles. It goes against everything they have been taught about pharmaceutical medication. With pharmaceutical, or with herbal medicine, the higher the dose, the stronger the effect and potency of the medicine.

Homeopathy is just the opposite. It is based on the Law of Similars, which means treat with a "like" or similar substance, rather than an opposite substance. An example of this Law would be vaccinations; using a small dose of a something to trigger the immune system to rally to prevent the disease. The great benefit of homeopathy, and using tiny doses to trigger healing, is that harmful side-effects are virtually non-existent.

Extreme dilution enhances the curative properties of the homeopathic remedy. The number behind the name of a homeopathic medicine describes to what degree the remedy has been diluted. Arnica is the most common homeopathic medicine used in the U.S. It is available in 6c or 30c or 200c strengths. This means that the substance, in this case a mountain flower, has been diluted and made potent, based on homeopathic methods that have been used since the 1700s when Dr. Samuel Hahnemann discovered them.

We are only beginning to understand the sub-atomic universe and how mighty tiny particles can be.

So, homeopathic HCG is a very diluted form of the HCG hormone. Remember that the human body does not always need a huge amount of something at any one time. Our cells are very tiny and a small amount of something that can be utilized readily is much better, and more effective, than a large amount of something that cannot be broken down enough to be used at a cellular level.

How to Know If You Are a Good Candidate for the Fat Fix Diet

The Homeopathic HCG drops and diet can be used by almost anyone to help them lose weight. In my office we have put people through the regimen from teens to seniors, in various states of health and obesity. Teenagers may need more food, and should not do the program while participating in a strenuous sports program. The FAT FIX DIET will often help acne clear up.

Most prescription medication and hormone replacement such as Thyroid medication does not seem to present any sort of a problem.

Of course, if you are on a medical program, you should check with your physician, just as you would concerning anything you might add or change while you are receiving medical care. Be sure to let your doctor know that you are taking a homeopathic dose of the HCG. (See the section "How Homeopathy Works" on "How Homeopathy Works" on page 18 before approaching your doctor.)

In practice I have found that patients who are taking multiple medications or have an underlying chronic health condition may have a little more difficulty adjusting to the HCG. Their weight loss may be slower. However, every single person in my practice who has done the program has lost weight. There are a few things I watch out for to make sure that someone will do well on the diet, without being hungry, and able to lose as much weight as possible:

- Low Function Thyroid
- Sluggish Gall Bladder
- Constipation

Very often, losing weight with the HCG method is going to help anyone who needs it to improve their health and their chronic conditions. One of my patients had a 40 point drop in cholesterol after a month on the HCG.

The fact that you are reducing the amount of starch and sugar you eat while on the HCG diet will lower your triglycerides and cholesterol because triglycerides and cholesterol are both made out of glucose or blood sugar.

Starches like flours, grains, breads, potatoes and white rice are broken down into sugars when they are digested. Along with refined sugars, the starches will spike blood sugar levels. The body has to prevent the sugar concentration in the blood from becoming too high or brain function is interrupted and nerves are affected. So the sugar is transported to the liver where it is converted into fatty acids called triglycerides. The triglycerides re-enter the blood for transportation to cells for fuel. Excess triglycerides travel back to the liver and are formed into cholesterol. Cholesterol is used to make sex hormones, and as lubrication for the body. Every cell has a protective fat envelope or sheath. So, cholesterol is not only vital for human health, it is also cancer protective, since it protects the cells. That is why lowering the cholesterol too much with prescription medication is a cancer risk, and studies do not show that statin cholesterol drugs have made a dent in heart disease. Since they also impair liver function there is a big risk for hardly any benefit.

Please note that the cholesterol may increase *during* the FAT FIX DIET program. The HCG is mobilizing your fat cells to release fat, so the circulating fat in the blood may increase temporarily. This may be reflected in any blood work. This is not dangerous because the body will only release the fat it can actually utilize, so you don't need to worry that it will deposit in arteries. So, have your cholesterol count measured before or after using HCG, but not during the Phase 2 diet.

Eating dietary fat like butter and olive oil is responsible for very little cholesterol, which is manufactured in the liver and is vital for human health. After all, sex hormones are made out of cholesterol!

I often have my patients fill out a health analysis so that I can predict any problems they may encounter. I will use the analysis later to trouble-shoot if someone reaches a plateau or does not lose as easily as expected. Sections of the analysis are reprinted in this manual so that you can see if you should add any supplements to help you get the most out of your program.

Thyroid: The first thing I look for is unidentified low thyroid. This means that the thyroid is not producing quite enough of one or more thyroid hormones, or the thyroid is not responding to hormones produced by other glands.

Many, many people, especially women, suffer from an undiagnosed hypo (low) thyroid condition. The thyroid hormone level may not be low enough to show up on a standard blood test because the purpose of the blood work is to identify thyroid disease that requires medical treatment. There is a large gap between disease and optimal function of the thyroid.

Low thyroid function is responsible for many miseries, including infertility, depression, weight gain, difficulty losing weight, sleep problems, and low body temperature.

The thyroid is dependent on iodine for function. Iodine is a mineral present in vegetables grown in soil rich in minerals. Iodine is found most abundantly in the sea and in sea vegetables. There are areas, particularly in mountainous regions far from iodine rich oceans, where there is so little iodine that brain function is affected. The medical term is "cretinism".

In the United States, there is a large "goiter belt" across the mid-West, where iodine is not present in the soil. Goiter is enlarged thyroid. Many glands and organs will get larger in size if they do not have the nutrients they need. The thyroid needs iodine to function. Iodine is also used by the immune system to kill bacteria in the blood.

By using natural thyroid support, which may include iodine, the thyroid can function better. The person may feel better, more energetic, happier and lose weight more easily.

LIVER/GALL BLADDER FUNCTION is the second thing I look for to ensure easier weight loss. The liver has over 200 functions. Not only is the liver the major detoxification organ in the body, but it also interacts with the hormonal system in the body.

Toxic by-products from the food we eat and the environment exit the liver in the bile. The gall bladder "catches" some of the bile and holds it until fat in the form of oil or butter is eaten. Then the gall bladder releases the bile so that the fat is emulsified, or broken down. You know how oil and water don't mix? If the oil is emulsified, it is broken down into tiny globs so that it will mix with the water.

The body needs to have emulsified or broken down bits of fat—fatty acids—as a nutrient. These essential fatty acids carry fat-soluble vitamins through the walls of the intestine into the lymph system to be carried to each cell in the body.

The bile that is stored in the gall bladder must be thin enough to easily flow when the gall bladder contracts. If the bile gets thick, like cream, and will not flow easily. Toxins not fully broken down in the liver may cause the bile to get thick, leading to congestion and stone formation. This slow, thick bile may interfere with the breakdown of fats. Some symptoms of this include nausea, excess appetite, migraine head-aches, hot flashes, constipation, joint stiffness and difficulty losing weight.

Gall stones are soft and seldom dangerous, but may be very uncomfortable. They can be released by doing a gall bladder cleanse. (See the back section for instructions on how to do this.)

Liver and gall bladder congestion is one of the reasons for weight problems; both weight gain and inability to lose readily.

During the HCG diet, because of the lack of dietary fat, the gall bladder will not empty as frequently. If the bile is already thick, this may aggravate gall bladder symptoms.

The remedy is to include some gall bladder support along with the program. See the section called *Supplements for Success* (page 25) for liver/gall bladder support.

CONSTIPATION: If constipation occurs during the HCG program, gall bladder/liver support is indicated and supplements supporting liver/gall bladder may help. Digestion and elimination is like a factory assembly line. Each step of the way must function in order to get an "end product"!

Probiotics and mild laxatives may also help to relieve constipation. Smooth Move Tea, available at your health food store, is an effective temporary solution. Magnesium supplements may be used, and you may try bathing in an Epsom Salts bath. Epsom Salts contain magnesium.

If constipation is a chronic problem, it may become worse during the HCG diet and mild laxatives may be included. Laxatives should not be relied on daily. Find a natural medicine practitioner who can find the root cause and help you remedy it. Elimination should be as natural as eating. Metabolism is an assembly line. Food is eaten, nutrients removed, and waste eliminated. If waste is building up inside the intestine, it is also leaking back into the blood and that can lead to a variety of chronic problems and eventual disease states.

To Get Started

There are only a few things you need to get started losing weight: decision, instructions, Homeopathic HCG and allowed foods organized for your life.

Decide that you are going to give the FAT FIX DIET Plan your best shot for 1-2 weeks. If you are sick and tired of carrying around a spare tire, looking and feeling less than your best, or you are worried about your health, this is the best thing you can do for yourself. No diet is always easy, but this plan is simple.

Even if you have failed at diets before, the FAT FIX DIET Plan will work for you. People who have been stuck for years at a weight that would not budge lose weight on this diet. Decide to follow the plan exactly for 1-2 weeks and see how you feel about the plan after that. You have nothing to lose but weight and fat.

Read all the "How To Do the Diet" instructions carefully and make sure you understand them. This book is constructed so that you can just follow along and do the diet to lose, or you can gain a more in-depth understanding of how the diet works. There is also information on what to do if you need to debug your loss if you get bogged along the way.

This book is a guide designed to help you get maximum success from your diet and reap all the health benefits of your new

Take care of your body. It's the only place you have to live.

Jim Rohn

shape. Watch how your body responds to the program and you understand how to keep the weight from coming back.

Look over the recipe ideas. Make sure you understand what foods are allowed and organize your life and eating so that you can eat according to the diet plan. It may look difficult, if you have been living on sandwiches, snack foods, fast food and pastries. But once you start taking the drops you will be surprised how easy the plan is.

If you eat out often, you can still follow the diet plan. Ask for steamed vegetables or plain salad, then add lemon juice or salsa for flavor. Add chicken, meat or fish and you have a meal.

Use a scale and/or tape measure to mark your progress. There is nothing like seeing the scale change to keep you motivated.

Have fun. Enjoy your food. Get someone to help you if you are not a cook and don't know how to make the recipes work for you. The Fat Fix Plan can become a new lifestyle. You will always be able to fall back on the Maintenance to keep yourself healthy and slim for the rest of your life.

Using the Fat Fix Diet HCG Program in My Practice

As a Naturopath and Nutritionist in Los Angeles, I have helped many people have success on the FAT FIX DIET Homeopathic HCG diet plan. I have made some modifications to the original Dr. Simeons diet to get people through as comfortably as possible while still experiencing substantial weight loss.

Most of my patients have done my version of the diet with great success. Weight loss of 20-25 pounds in a month or six weeks is common, if that much weight loss is needed. Others who did not need to lose that much weight, including myself, have lost 8-10 pounds easily. If more weight loss is desired, further rounds of the entire HCG program are done.

Another good reducing exercise consists in placing both hands against the table edge and pushing back.

Robert Quillen

Because I have helped so many people lose weight successfully, I have learned how to debug problems that may cause slow or stuck pounds from coming off.

This book was written so that others could achieve success, as well. There are other books on the HCG program, but few are written by Naturopaths[1] or Nutritionists who understand the body well enough to assess for underlying conditions that may keep a person from losing quickly and comfortably.

---

1   Naturopath: a holistic health practitioner trained to use non-drug, Nature-based remedies to help the body heal and repair.

I have also changed the eating plan, based on my years of experience helping people balance their blood sugar levels so that they can lose weight, and avoid many chronic conditions. Before I heard about the HCG weight loss plan, I considered blood sugar issues (hypoglycemia, pre-Diabetes, and Diabetes Type II) as the biggest health challenge of our times. Our "modern" diseases of cancer and heart disease can be traced to the increased consumption of simple carbohydrates like white flour and white sugar. Processed oils, manufactured fats like margarine, and high temperature fried foods are another factor, along with the artificial flavors and chemicals that comprise so much of the American diet.

The eating regimen that I recommend for the FAT FIX DIET program allows for more protein and vegetables than the original 500 calorie per day diet. When Dr. A.T.W. Simeons did his research in the Italy of the 1950s, the world was a different place. Italians took a siesta daily for 2 hours after lunch. The food was much more nutrient-dense than our modern farming practices produce now. People lived in family settings, and walked more and lived less stressful lives.

In contrast, many of my patients work in the television industry, with very long hours and high stress environment. Others commute great distances on Los Angeles freeways.

Every single person who has actually done my FAT FIX DIET program has lost a great deal of weight. People lose as much as Dr. Simeons suggests as the maximum that should be lost in a 4-6 week period.

My interest in this program was not only to help people lose weight, but to lose it in the healthiest way. Weight loss is not a goal in itself, for a Nutritionist. But weight loss should be a by-product of a healthier life style and eating regimen. I have not seen any health issues created by the homeopathic HCG, only health benefits. Any symptoms that appear mean there is an underlying condition.

The Debug section is designed to help you handle anything that might come up. Most people sail through the Fat Fix Diet, lose weight easily, and are thrilled with the results.

The Fat Fix Diet program supplies the key ingredients for people to lose weight successfully and keep it off, and improve their health at the same time.

The original diet is also presented here, as Dr. Simeons wrote it, for those who feel more comfortable following his original work. If you have been using this approach, and it has worked for you, feel free to continue. However, the Debug information in this manual may help you get even more out of your diet and handle any snags you may encounter. And the recipes will make the food more pleasurable.

If you are concerned about eating so little food on Dr. Simeons' diet, I suggest that you give my program a try. There is no calorie counting, but healthy amounts of protein, fruits and vegetables. It has worked for hundreds of people who needed to lose weight, either a substantial amount, or a small amount.

Because of the greater variety allowed in my program, many find that they can stick to the diet longer because they are enjoying their food more. Also, greater variety in choices may translate into more nutrients, so it may be healthier in the long run.

Here are the benefits to using the Homeopathic HCG with the FAT FIX DIET Plan:

- No painful injections or prescriptions
- No need to send away for prescription HCG from foreign countries
- Homeopathic HCG made at an FDA certified American Laboratory
- Less expense
- More food to satisfy you and easier transition back to "normal" eating
- Same great results of fast weight loss
- Dramatic loss of inches and stored fat
- Better, more restful sleep
- More energy
- Disappearance or reduction of aches and pains
- Freedom from food cravings and addictions

The main point about both Dr. Simeons' diet and mine is that insulin levels stay balanced and low. Dr. Simeons used the calorie deprivation approach and my approach is balanced blood sugar. Stable blood sugar allows the HCG to do its seeming magic and stimulate the fat cells to let go of fat.

The result is not only loss of weight, but less inflammation, bloat and swelling. Patients also report better sleep and some have significant pain relief. Metabolism is improved, so that you burn food more efficiently in the future and do not gain weight as easily.

Your body is reshaped. Some people report that their body takes on a better shape than they ever had in their lives. The loss of inches and fat from deposits that make the body look misshapen is one of the greatest benefits. Only with vigorous physical exercise, along with dieting, have I seen the body shape become so attractive. Since only moderate or mild exercise is recommended, this is one of the happiest benefits of the FAT FIX DIET program.

Reduce, Reshape and Reset. That is what can be expected on the FAT FIX DIET program.

Why My Program is Different From the Original

If you have read the original manuscript from Dr. Simeons, who developed the prescription HCG diet, you will notice that my diet is different. I have done a lot of research on weight loss over the past few years, and I have applied what I have learned.

Many of the people in my practice work in the television and movie business. They work very long hours and needed a diet that would work for them.

The original Simeons diet was developed in Italy in the 1950s. There is a world of difference between Italy then and Los Angeles, or the United States, now. The quality of the food in Italy was probably much better and more nutritious, and the lifestyle would have been much slower and less stressful.

My program is still low calorie, but not just 500 calories like the original. I added more protein, more vegetables, and even more fruit. People who are keeping very long hours at work or staying up late at night may even need more protein. See the section on Blood Sugar (page 63) for a more complete explanation.

Never Count Calories—Count the Inches You Lose!

We're the country that has more food to eat than any other country in the world, and with more diets to keep us from eating it.

Author Unknown

Wouldn't anyone lose weight on so few calories per day?

Yes, most would. But they would not lose weight from the same places as they would while on the HCG diet, and they would be hungry, if not starving. One of the amazing things about the HCG drops is that you lose weight where you want to lose it, because it mobilizes the fat that is just storage, and not fat that is there for contour. People don't lose in their face and thinner parts first, and the fat places last, as can happen on usual diets. Also, there is little hunger on this diet, especially after the first couple of days. You might feel a little "empty", especially if you skip meals. It is important to eat regularly, even breaking up the allowed food so that you eat every 2-3 hours. You will lose inches on this program and feel "sleeker".

On the HCG program you are stimulating the body to let go of fat from the fat cells. Although you are eating low calorie, you are accessing 1500 of your own fat calories per day. That is why you should expect to feel good, and lose fast. As far as I know, no other diet can make your own fat cells break down as fast.

The original diet says to skip breakfast and only drink tea or coffee. Yours is different. Why?

I found that many people could not really skip breakfast completely, depending on their lifestyle and schedule. Eating some protein for breakfast does not seem to stop weight loss. I don't know why coffee is allowed, except for the fact that the doctor who did the research was Italian! (Hence the bread sticks, as well.) Those who dislike breakfast may wait until lunch to eat. However, in general, skipping breakfast is not a healthy practice. This diet, and all weight management, is all about stable blood sugar and low/stable insulin levels.

Skipping breakfast means that your blood sugar dips too low. If you are not hungry in the morning, this may mean that your blood sugar is really out of synch and you may be eating too much at night. If this is the case, after the diet be sure to eat some protein and fat for breakfast.

What happens if I cheat or have to go to an event where I cannot stick to the diet?

You may find that you do gain back a couple of pounds. Just keep going. If you have any issues, like cravings or hunger, there are tricks you can use.

For one thing, be sure to prepare appetizing food, using the recipe ideas. Adding spices and lemon and garlic can go a long way towards helping you enjoy your meals. I use a George Foreman grill that will cook steak, chicken, fish,— even veggies, in just a few minutes. The fat runs off into a tray and the food is delicious. Being organized is very important so that you are not confronted with a need to eat fast with no healthy options. Sugar cravings may be a sign that you have an imbalance of good bugs in the intestine, so taking probiotics may help. Your intestine has trillions of helpful critters that digest your food, make vitamins for you and keep your intestine working properly. Antibiotics, sugar, white flour, other drugs and medicines, eating all cooked foods instead of raw or fermented foods, can deplete the good bugs of what they need to survive. Just like in a garden, you cannot sterilize the soil and then grow flowers or vegetables. When the good bugs start dying off, the opportunistic bugs start multiplying. They feed off the gut, but offer nothing in return.

Your intestine is like a neighborhood. Keep it in good repair and good neighbors will move in. Let it become derelict and the crack dealers set up operations.

Probiotics, acidophilus and bifidus and many other organisms that help replace the good bugs are helpful if you do not eat perfectly (who does?) or have ever taken antibiotics.

Gas and bloating, diarrhea or constipation, may be signs that you need more good bugs.

Sweet cravings may be helped by eating cinnamon, which helps balance your blood sugar, so bake some apples with cinnamon, nutmeg and stevia.

Should I take vitamins while on the diet?

No one needs less nutrients generally. There may be imbalances, with certain nutrients consumed in greater quantity than needed, and others undersupplied. But no one eating a Western diet gets enough of all nutrients needed by the body. *Even organic produce does not have the same amount of nutrients it had 80 years ago.*

Synthetic vitamins, manufactured in chemical laboratories, may be taken in doses that are too high and thus create more imbalances. Notice that single vitamins never exist in Nature, but are always combined with other vitamins, minerals, enzymes.

That is why I like Standard Process™ Whole Food supplements. Standard Process supplements are available through practitioners only. You can check the company website at www.standardprocess.com for an office near you that carries the supplements. If you live outside the U.S.A., check with your local distributor for substitute supplements.

You can take *Cyrofood* or *Catalyn* or *Fortil B-12* for a multi-vitamin. Cyrofood also has calcium. You may want to take *Cataplex B* (*Cataplex G* if you have high blood pressure), which are the B complex products. Take *Zypan* and/or *Multizyme* if you have stomach/digestive issues. You need to be sure to digest the protein you are eating.

If you have a history of gall bladder problems, I suggest you take 6-8 *AF Betafood* or *Betafood* while on the diet. Eating no-fat food can aggravate the gall bladder because it needs dietary fat to "purge" or empty itself. *Zymex* is very good if you tend towards intestinal gas or bloating. Skip fish oils and other oil-based supplements while you are on the Phase 2 diet, then add them back in on the Phase 3 Maintenance. Some people may experience some leg cramps on the diet. If this is the case, increase your water intake. You may also add some magnesium and/or potassium supplements, Magnesium Lactate or Organic Minerals.

It is always best to take "food source" vitamins. Most of the vitamins sold in stores, even health food stores, are synthetic. That means they were made in the laboratory, not made by Nature. Some will tell you that there is no difference. However, consider that most commercially sold B vitamins are made from coal tar! Some B vitamins are even manufactured in the same factories that make coal tar.

I have a great diet. You're allowed to eat anything you want, but you must eat it with naked fat people.

Ed Bluestone

Actually, it is not the tar itself that is put in B vitamins, but a derivative. But it is still nothing like the B vitamins that are in real food. For one thing, there are probably B vitamins that we have not discovered yet. But synthetic B's only contain a few vitamins that are easily and cheaply thrown together.

Meat, fruits and dairy products all contain B vitamins, as well as grains and cereals. White flour and white rice are stripped of B vitamins. Brown color in bread does not mean it is made from good quality wheat, just as molasses can be used to dye white sugar brown. B12, and important nutrient for mental health, is found only in animal products. Organic eggs are a good source of B12.

Vitamins are "vital" to the body because they are needed for the processes that take place on a cellular level as helpers to the hundreds of activities performed by every kind of cell in the body.

So, don't waste your money on cheap, inferior vitamins. Your body will pee out 50-90% of synthetic vitamins. And many multi-vitamins have a thick coating so that the stomach acid will not destroy them before they can reach the intestine. Listen for the sound of that vitamin pinging against the wall of your toilet! Yes, many will pass straight through the intestine—a very expensive form of fiber.

More Benefits To The Fat Fix Diet Program

As a Naturopath, it was very important to me to find a program that made people healthier, while they lost weight. There are sick skinny people, so girth is not a measure of health.

As the successes started pouring in, many people reported additional benefits from the FAT FIX DIET program.

Aches and pains disappeared from joints. Head-aches stopped. Acne cleared up. Increased energy and better sleep were reported. Indigestion, bloating and gas disappeared. Hot flashes and PMS were improved.

High Blood pressure often decreases or normalizes and people may find they need to coordinate with their medical doctor to reduce their blood pressure medication. Note also that the Whey Protein Shake recommended for breakfast on the FAT FIX DIET may help reduce high blood pressure, according to studies.

Patients have reported significant drops in cholesterol. Cholesterol medication interferes with the production of liver enzymes in order to suppress production of cholesterol. This is not the healthiest thing for your liver, and that is why liver enzyme tests must be ordered twice a year when people are taking cholesterol-lowering drugs. The natural way to reduce cholesterol is to cut back on sugar and grains. The

The leading cause of death among fashion models is falling through street grates.

Dave Barry

41

liver makes cholesterol out of excess blood sugar, not out of fat. So, the eating plan on the FAT FIX DIET program is the best thing for your cholesterol. And avoiding cholesterol medication is the best thing for your liver, the major organ that detoxifies the body and filters your blood.

Chronic symptoms that people had considered a part of ageing, or just how their body was, often cleared up or lessened. Painkillers, sleeping medications and other drugs were not needed as much.

Blood sugar levels often drop and less insulin may be needed for Diabetics. Diabetics should monitor their blood sugar closely on the FAT FIX DIET.

Is it the HCG or the Eating Plan?

Body fat apparently takes on a life of its own. It produces hormones, particularly estrogen, which may be a cancer risk. Fat interacts with the other glands, such as the adrenals, and pancreas, and receives hormonal messages that seem to keep the fat stuck.

Getting rid of excess body fat seems to calm down the endocrine system so that the hormones are more balanced. This means that the hormones are operating more steadily, without wild fluctuations that affect your emotions too dramatically. For example, feeling sad and weepy before a period is not uncommon for a woman when her progesterone level drops suddenly during her menstrual cycle. And hormones can make a man or woman act out sexual behavior that can be delightful—or devastating—to their relationships.

So, shrinking the amount of excess fat has many benefits, other than purely cosmetic. Toxins store in the body fat, and mobilizing the fat from the cells means that you are melting down your toxic load while you are melting down your hips and belly.

But the HCG won't work without you changing how you are eating. You must get rid of the sugars and starches. When the body has less sugar in the blood, insulin levels stay low. And that is the time when the Homeopathic HCG will work. The action of HCG is the opposite of insulin. To put it very simply, insulin is a fat "growing" hormone and HCG is a fat "shrinking" hormone. But HCG will not work if the insulin level is high—they cancel each other out.

Insulin is released when the sugar and starch from our food enters the bloodstream following a meal or snack. Lower the insulin levels by cutting out sugars and grains, take the HCG drops, and the body responds beautifully.

The HCG may seem to work like Magic, but the way it works in the body is pure science.

Cravings disappear on the HCG, and most people report they enjoy eating this new way. At least most of the time!

The Fat Fix Diet with Magic Drops™

How To Do the Diet

Read these instructions carefully and make sure you completely understand them. Your success depends on following the instructions. This diet really works—if you do it correctly.

Weigh yourself every day during the diet and maintenance programs, first thing in a.m., no clothes. Keep a log of weight daily.

Plan your schedule for Phase 1 Binge Days, Phase 2 Diet Days and Phase 3 Maintenance Days. Choose a program for 3 weeks, 4 weeks or 6 weeks.

There is a charm about the forbidden that makes it unspeakably desirable.

Mark Twain

Phase 1: Days 1 and 2 — Bingeing

Take 12 drops 3 times per day. Take the drops first thing in the morning and then on schedule, spacing them a few hours apart throughout the day. Hold the drops under the tongue for a three or four minutes so they have a chance to be absorbed. Swallow any remaining. Do not put anything in your mouth 15 minutes before or after taking the drops. This includes water and brushing your teeth. The drops are basically flavorless.

skip?

MRC Protein
or
Collagen Peptides

If you are using the Magic Drops HCG sublingual pellets, dispense 5 pellets into the cap of the bottle. Try not to touch with your fingers. Drop the pellets from the cap under your tongue and let them dissolve. They taste slightly sweet and very pleasant.

These first two day are Binge Days. Binge means "indulge excessively". Eat lots of fattening food all day long, including fried and creamy foods. Cheeseburgers, pizza, ice cream, donuts, French fries, etc. You may also eat healthier fats like avocado and sour cream. You must do this to jump-start the fat loss!! The bingeing seems to help the body give up fat when you start the next phase of the FAT FIX DIET program.

Do not skip this step! You will be hungrier if you do.

Many people actually lose weight on the binge days. Other people will gain a pound or two. Either is normal. If you gain, do not worry, as the extra couple of pounds will be rapidly lost when you start the next Phase.

Phase 2

Choose to do a 3-week, 4-week or 6-week program. Follow the Phase 2 eating plan strictly every day for the number to weeks you choose.

One bottle of Magic Drops will last you 4 weeks, if you measure the drops carefully. You will need 2 bottles if you choose a 6-week program. One bottle of Magic Drops Homeopathic HCG pellets will last you 5–6 weeks.

What To Eat

Drinks lots of pure water, filtered or spring, up to a ½ gallon per day.

Don't worry too much about the amount of calories you eat. Generally speaking avoid all processed and refined foods. Stick to the basic diet of protein, vegetables and some fruit and your calories will be low enough. Don't eat too much protein at a time. Eat regularly during the day, don't skip meals, and keep your blood sugar balanced. That will allow the Magic Drops to help trigger fat burning hormones so you utilize your own body fat for fuel.

BREAKFAST: You may skip breakfast, but you may also have a light protein breakfast. You may have an egg white omelet (with a vegetable) or a shake of whey powder, berries, and water. Do not use Soy protein, as many people are allergic to soy and it may suppress thyroid. Use a whey protein powder that has nothing else in it, except whey protein.[1] Standard Process makes the best Whey Protein called Whey Pro Complete. You may use Stevia[2] to sweeten your shake. Flavored stevia may be used, such as chocolate or vanilla cream. (Find recipe ideas in Recipe section.)

TEA OR COFFEE: Drink in any quantity of tea or coffee without sugar or artificial sweeteners. Stevia may be used. 1 tablespoon of milk (not cream) is allowed in 24 hour period. Herbal tea and naturally sparkling water may be used. Try adding flavored Stevia (Sweet Leaf brand) or lemon or lime

---

1 Whey is a milk protein. The liquid that separates from the solids in yogurt is whey.

2 Stevia is made from a South American plant. It tastes sweet, but does not contain sugar or calories, and is not artificial. No diet or artificial products may be used on the diet.

juice to sparkling water. No "diet" drinks may be used. Splenda may not be used.

LUNCH 6 oz. of veal, beef, chicken breast, white fish, lobster, crab or shrimp. All visible fat must be removed and meat broiled or grilled in no fat.

steam

VEGETABLES from following list, or from the extended list:

Spinach, chard, chicory, beet greens, green salad (no dressing except lemon juice), tomatoes, celery, fennel, onions, red radishes, cucumbers, asparagus, cabbage.

Additional vegetables allowed:

Bamboo shoots, bean sprouts, beet greens, bok choy greens, broccoli, cauliflower, celery, collard greens, endive, escarole, garlic, kale, kohlrabi, lettuces, mushrooms, mustard greens, parsley, radishes, raw cob corn, spinach, string beans, summer squashes, turnip greens, watercress, yellow squash, zucchini squash.

Drain

One bread stick *or* one Melba toast *or* one medium whole grain cracker.

Fruit

An apple, orange or a handful of strawberries or other berries or one-half grapefruit. No mango, watermelon or banana or other tropical fruits. *pineapple*

DINNER: Same choices as lunch. The fruits and/or bread sticks may be eaten between meals for a snack. Eat different protein for lunch and dinner. Try not to eat anything after 8 p.m.

Snack

Don't skip meals, don't save all your food for later in the day and don't let yourself get too hungry between meals. You may break your meals up into 5-6 meals a day, if you need to, in order not to get hungry.

You may use 1 cup skim cottage cheese (organic is best) 2 times per week. More often if you are vegetarian and not using meat or chicken. Too much dairy may slow weight loss. Plain yogurt may also be used for vegetarians.

check

Salt, pepper, marjoram, thyme, mustard powder, garlic, basil, parsley, etc, may be used for seasoning, but no oil or butter.

Allowed fish is real fish, not imitation fish. You may choose flounder, haddock, ling cod, monkfish, pike, orange roughy, cod, bass, sole, snapper, whiting, turbot, cisco, grouper. No tuna, salmon or oily fish, or pickled or dried fish.

Some fat is good ?

It is a hard matter, my fellow citizens, to argue with the belly, since it has no ears.

Plutarch

Hitting a Plateau

If you hit a plateau for 3 days and don't lose, you may have 6 large apples with no other food for one day. It is not unusual to hit a plateau after 10-14 days. You may stop losing for 3 or even 4 days. Just hang in there and keep doing the diet or do the apple day. You will lose again. You may also try taking an extra dose of drops. Weight still not budging after an apple day? Try taking 1 teaspoon of butter or nut butter, virgin olive oil or raw coconut oil at bedtime. Don't overdo this remedy!

You can try cutting back on fruit to break a stall. Try eating just protein and vegetables for a couple of days. Also, see the section on creams and lotions below, and eliminate any you may be using.

Consider eliminating all dairy for a few days. Some people have a hidden dairy intolerance and removing even the tablespoon of milk allowed in coffee may break the plateau for sensitive individuals. Note: eggs are not dairy.

Still Hungry

Some people report feeling more "empty" than hungry. If you find yourself unbearably hungry between meals, try saving some protein for a snack and eating smaller, more frequent meals. You may have some extra vegetables, too. An extra dose of the homeopathic HCG may be taken.

People who stay up very late report being more hungry. Try to keep a regular schedule and get to bed before midnight, if possible. You may find you need some extra sleep on the program. The balanced blood sugar on the HCG program may help you sleep better! Also, you may need some gall bladder supplements while taking the drops. Ask us about using Homeopathic Appetite control.

Menstrual Cycle

Women may experience a temporary weight gain while on the program just before their period has begun. Usually the weight will drop again a couple of days after the period starts. If you normally experience weight gain or bloating, you may expect this. Do not do anything unusual, but eat strictly according to the regular plan of protein, fruits and veggies. It is best not to start the program just before your period, but wait until afterwards.

Skin Creams and Lotions

It is advised that only non-oily moisturizer may be used. Alba makes a non-oily moisturizer-available at Health Food Stores. Amazon.com has other oil free moisturizers. Aveeno has a body lotion and is available in drug stores. Tate's Conditioner is made from organic plant ingredients and is a good choice.

Some women are able to use light creams. If weight loss is stalled, consider not using creams at all for a few days to see if this is the reason.

Diet Drinks, Gum and Mints

No diet drinks of any kind are allowed. No chemical or processed foods of any kind. No gum or mints except those with Xylitol or Stevia may be used.

Exercise

Only mild to moderate exercise is recommended. Don't do extreme exercise or hard workouts that may make you hungrier.

Phase 3—Maintenance

Key to Keeping the Weight Off

It is vital that you follow this 3 week program after your weight loss program is finished. This will reset your metabolism and prevent gaining the weight back.

Increase your calorie and portion intake. You may add back *gradually* in dairy, nuts, cheese and oil. Stick to good oils like butter, olive and coconut oil or other unrefined oils.

Absolutely no sugars of any kind—no honey, corn syrup, *Stevia (OK) + Xylitol* molasses, dextrose, sucrose, etc. Read labels to watch for hidden sugars. Avoid packaged and processed foods.

Eat the same types of proteins, fruits and vegetables, but increase quantities.

Eat the same types of proteins, fruits and vegetables, but increase quantities.

No starch—no bread, pasta, pastries, rice, potatoes, white or brown. You may continue eating the 2 bread sticks or Melba toast per day.

No artificial sweeteners. No fast food.

No trans fats (fried or processed fats) or nitrites (sausage or deli meats).

It is important that you add healthy fats back into your diet on the Maintenance and when you are finished with the program. Real (organic) butter, unrefined oils like olive, walnut, peanut, safflower oils, raw coconut oil, and raw ground nut butters are good choices. Fish oil, Evening Primrose oil and Wheat Germ oil can all be taken as supplements. All your cells, including brain and nerve cells, need these oils and your skin and hair will get very dry if you don't add back in good fats.

If You Need to Lose More Weight

Each time you do Phases 1, 2 and 3 is called a "Round". You can start a second Round as soon as you are ready. If you wait to do a second Round, be sure to stay on the Maintenance to avoid gaining back any weight.

If you decide to do a third Round, it is a good idea to wait 5-6 weeks between Phase 3 (Maintenance) and starting a new Phase 1 (Binge). That helps the Magic Drops Homeopathic HCG to be more active in your body. See the next section for advice on maintaining your weight. If appetite is a problem, there is homeopathic appetite control available.

Forever After—How to Maintain Your Lower Weight

As long as your weight does not go up more than 2 pounds, stick to what you are doing. If weight goes up 2 pounds, you can try this: skip breakfast and lunch, but drink plenty of water. For dinner eat a huge steak with an apple or tomato (raw) and nothing else. You may also divide the steak into 2-3 servings and eat during the day if you cannot fast all day until dinner. Other protein choices seem to work, as well.

Or you can just eat protein and vegetables and a little fat for one or two days. Eat only 1-2 tablespoons of fat, eat protein 2-3 meals. Avoid all starches, grains, breads, pastas and sugars. You should lose the weight again quickly by doing this. So, stay on top of your weight. If you gain more than two pounds, handle it immediately before your body has a chance to set itself at a higher weight. *Back to Ph 2—*

> Food is like sex: when you abstain, even the worst stuff begins to look good.
>
> **Beth McCollister**

Recommended Supplements

The supplements recommended come from Standard Process.™

Cyrofood or *Catalyn* for multivitamin and minerals.

Many people need support for the liver/gall bladder while on the diet. If you have any history of gall bladder problems or stones, or if you have had gall bladder surgery, be sure to use gall bladder supplements such as *AF Betafood, Betafood, Cholacol, Choline, Cholaplex*. Cholacol in particular is indicated for people who have had their gall bladder removed. A herb called Milk Thistle is also beneficial for the liver.

You may take whole B vitamins such as *Cataplex B or Cataplex B12* for energy.

Digestive enzymes are also a good idea. It is important that you digest all the protein and nutrients you will be eating on the program. Take *Zypan* for protein digestion and/or *Multizyme* or *Enzycore* for digestion of protein and carbohydrates, including fruits and vegetables. Digestive enzymes may also be protective against diabetes and cancer.

Many people with a history of weight problems have an underactive or low function thyroid. This may or may not show up on blood tests, but thyroid function is vital for general health and metabolism. See the Thyroid (page 79) and Adrenal (page 81) sections of this manual.

Take *Thytrophin* for non-hormonal thyroid support. Thytrophin may also help your thyroid medication work better, if you are taking medication. Thytrophin is very helpful if there is any history of depression.

Take *Drenatrophin* or *Drenamin* for adrenal support. Fatigue or history of anxiety are indications of adrenal burn-out. Magnesium and iodine are two minerals that many people are deficient in. Both may be supplemented to help with weight loss and general health.

Happily Ever After

After your hard work and sacrifice has paid off, and you have a new shape, and your clothes are loose, or you are swanking a new outfit, what then?

One of the most common questions I get is, "When do I get to go back to my usual way of eating?" The answer is, "That depends."

It depends a lot on whether you want to keep your body the way it is after you have attained your ideal weight. If you do, then you probably can never go back to your old ways. After all, that is how you gained unwanted pounds and that roll of blubber in the first place!

Can you eat bread and dessert? Occasionally. Eat it every day, and you will gain back. Whether you gain quickly or slowly depends on you.

First of all, do the Maintenance strictly. That will really set your weight loss. Many people who don't follow the Maintenance regain at least some weight, and have to start again. If they stick to the Maintenance after their second try, they report that the weight does stabilize.

I do consider the Maintenance a pretty ideal way to eat for most people. Some people naturally have a higher tolerance for starchy carbs than others. Men often can eat more starch than women because they have more muscle mass, and that increases their metabolism. But men are becoming Diabetic

> She looked as if she had been poured into her clothes and had forgotten to say "when."
> **P.G. Wodehouse**

at a higher rate than women. The Maintenance diet is the perfect anti-Diabetes, anti-Cancer, anti-high blood pressure, anti-high cholesterol, anti-obesity diet.

Gain→ help →

- So, add grains, breads and pastas, and desserts back in very slowly after the Phase 2 Maintenance. If you gain even a smidge of weight—2 pounds—do a steak or protein day.

Or go back on the Maintenance diet for a few days.

If you use the Maintenance diet as your basic stable eating regimen, you cannot go wrong. People do not need to eat grains at all. Many healthy cultures do not have any grains in their diet, natively. We all know those rare individuals who are able to eat anything and never gain a pound. But the majority of people are watching their weight carefully or struggling constantly to lose the extra weight they are carrying. Most of us cannot eat a diet of "crapohydrates",[1] carbs, sugars, pastries and processed chemical foods, and be either slim or healthy.

Forever Plan →

Eat the Maintenance diet most of the time and eat grains or desserts once a week, and you will be on your way to a lifetime of sleek good health.

To lose weight overnight Dr. Simeons recommended fasting all day and eating a huge steak and an apple or tomato at dinner.

I have seen any kind of protein work, and you can eat some protein at every meal, plus the apple or tomato at night. And the weight will come off.

You can balance the splurges of parties or celebrations with a protein day, and know that you can enjoy life without fear of packing on the pounds.

---

1   Crapohydrates—a term coined by Dr. Michael Dobbins, D.C.

But don't forget to eat a generally healthy diet of lots of fresh fruits and vegetables, and moderate amounts of protein, and excellent quality fats like virgin, cold pressed oils and some organic dairy on a regular basis. For more information on the benefit of raw dairy products see www.westonaprice.org.

Dietary fat is not the enemy. You lost the weight because of eliminating the carbs and sugars. Good quality fats will help you feel satisfied and balance your blood sugar, so they will contribute to your long term weight goals, as well as benefiting your general health, and protecting you against cancer and ageing disorders like Alzheimer's and Parkinson's.

Many people who have become junk food junkies, addicted to chemicals and artificial flavors, high fat, sugar and sodium, find they enjoy real food. And the difference in how their body responds to the real food is a revelation. And your wallet may benefit, also, as your health improves and you need less medical intervention.

Health is like a bank account. You need to deposit more than you withdraw. Nutrients from food are the currency needed to keep you "rich" in energy and well-being.

Appetite Control for the Maintenance Phase

Many people are concerned with what will happen when they stop the homeopathic HCG for the Maintenance Phase.

Often in the first couple of days the appetite is reduced. Your body is accustomed to less food and smaller portions. Some people even find they do not want to eat more, but it is important to increase your calories, and add in healthy fats.

Be sure not to cheat during the Maintenance Phase. You will not only regain weight, but your metabolism will not get reset, and you may trigger intense cravings for sugar and junk foods.

Eat frequently enough to keep your blood sugar stable. Use Whey Protein shakes as snacks for appetite control. Add raw coconut oil or flax oil to your shakes for good fats that stabilize appetite and blood sugar.

Increase your serving sizes and add virgin oils to your salads. Keep eating plenty of vegetables and green salads for bulk and nutrition.

There is a homeopathic appetite control that may be used for the Maintenance and Forever After phases. Check with a homeopathic practitioner or your distributor or with my office or website.

Continue on your supplements for liver/gall bladder, thyroid or adrenals. You may need additional supplementation for blood sugar, such as *Inositol* or *Paraplex* from Standard Process.

This way you have a system that you can use to help you achieve your ideal weight and then maintain the healthy weight for a lifetime.

Cravings and Our Chemical World

Sugar, chocolate, bread, ice cream, chips. Cheap, readily available, and even mood-altering. We are surrounded by foods that titillate our taste buds and soothe our jagged nerves (more coffee, anyone?), but also pile on pounds.

These foods may also have a nasty kick. After the initial lift, they drop us flat again when our blood sugar drops. Then the cycle of wanting these comfort foods starts over again. Give in to it and you may find yourself a junk-food junkie, with hardly any real food left in your diet at all.

Add in all the chemicals in our environment from industry and agriculture, and the chemicals in prescription medication. What is left is a giant science experiment with us as the guinea pigs.

Have you noticed the odd distribution of fat that some people have these days? The skinny forearms and bulbous upper arms, doughy loaves of thighs and bubble butts? These are probably caused by chemicals. With all the chemically created food cheaply available, some people are hardly eating any "real" food any more. Strawberry flavoring is not made from strawberries. It is made in a laboratory and designed to fool our taste buds into thinking it is eating strawberries. There is nothing healthy or helpful in these

It would be far easier to lose weight permanently if replacement parts weren't so handy in the refrigerator.

Hugh Allen

59

chemical flavorings, artificial sweeteners or fat substitutes like margarine. They are Frankenstein foods and cause our cells to make Frankenstein bodies.

Chemicals from food and industry can disrupt hormones, and make us eat more than we want to or need to. In fact, some snack foods may be chemically engineered to keep you eating more, just as cigarettes have addictive chemicals added. So, don't just blame your lack of willpower. You may be under some powerful influences.

You can help kick a drug or alcohol habit by stopping cold turkey. You can't stop eating, certainly, but you can kick the chemical habit.

One of the greatest benefits to the FAT FIX DIET program is that you are eating unprocessed foods. This is the time to discover organic and free range. Many people find themselves free of cravings for the first time ever. The human body is very susceptible to habits. Eating natural, farm raised foods can become a new habit that has enormous health benefits.

The result that you may be seeking the most is the loss of pounds and re-sculpting of the body. But don't be surprised if you find that other health conditions that you considered chronic or "normal" start to drop away.

Often there are big changes in the first week or two.

You can be free of sugar and junk food cravings and enjoy delicious, nourishing foods. And you can feel better, as well as look better.

Why You Need to
Get Enough Sleep

It is well known that sleep, or lack of it, can affect your ability to lose weight.

Some of the sleep deprivation is simply habit: staying up too late to watch TV or surf the Web or work late.

Sleep is as natural to the body as breathing or eating. If you try to sleep and cannot, there is something out of balance in the body.

The cardiologist's diet: If it tastes good, spit it out.

Anon

The good news is that the Magic Drops homeopathic HCG may help you to sleep better. Balancing your blood sugar, eliminating wheat and dairy products, and eating less food may calm down inflammation and give your internal organs a much needed rest.

While you are on the drops and the Maintenance program, try to get enough sleep. Regard this time as a spa program, and help your body by turning out the lights at an early hour. They don't call it "Beauty Sleep" for nothing!

Read on for information about the scientific studies about sleep.

Last year, a study showed that people who get an average of less than six hours of sleep each night are more than four times more likely to develop blood sugar dysfunction compared to those who average more than six hours per night.

And that may explain the results of another recent study from the UK. Researchers at the University of Warwick reviewed 16 sleep studies from various countries, including the U.S., Europe, and East Asia. Two results emerged: 1) Habitual lack of sleep increases risk of premature death by more than 10 percent, and 2) Excessive sleep (an average of more than nine hours each night) is also linked with premature death.

The difference: Too little sleep causes poor health, while too much sleep indicates that a serious health issue (such as hypertension) is already underway.[1]

In a recent study, researchers from Leiden University in the Netherlands checked the insulin levels of nine healthy people after eight hours of sleep. In the second phase of the study, the same subjects slept four hours and their insulin levels were checked again. Results showed that just this ONE night of inadequate sleep reduced insulin sensitivity by as much as 25 percent in some subjects.[2]

In the *Journal of Clinical Endocrinology & Metabolism*, the authors note that insulin sensitivity is apparently not fixed. Even in healthy people, a single night of poor sleep can temporarily knock everything out of whack.

Insulin hormone is a major factor in losing weight. So, it is also a factor in the FAT FIX DIET or in using any type of HCG. When the cells are insulin "sensitive" they will accept sugar inside to be burned for fuel and this lowers the blood

1   "Short Sleep Increases Risk of Death and Over-Long Sleep Can Indicate Serious Illness" Science Daily, 5/4/10, sciencedaily.com

2   "A Single Night of Partial Sleep Deprivation Induces Insulin Resistance in Multiple Metabolic Pathways in Healthy Subjects" Journal of Clinical Endocrinology & Metabolism, Published online ahead of print 4/6/10, jcem.endojournals.org

sugar levels. If too much sugar is circulating in the blood, the liver is prompted to make more triglycerides and that raises cholesterol levels and eventually that makes more fat tissue.

Lack of sleep is a cause for stalls and plateaus on the FAT FIX DIET. So, arrange your schedule so that you can get plenty of sleep while you are trying to lose weight.

What Is Stopping You From Getting A Good Night's Sleep?

I have helped many, many people sleep better over years of clinical practice. The good news is that sleep problems are not just about "stress", so there is something you can do about it. Sleeping well is the most natural thing in the world! If you cannot sleep, there is usually something going on physically—something that can be fixed.

The following are the main barriers I have found to a good night's sleep:

THYROID PROBLEMS. The thyroid hormones can be out of balance and that may cause heart palpitations at night. Or the body may not be able to relax enough to sleep. Have your thyroid checked by a practitioner who really understands about the thyroid. Many doctors do not know how to test correctly for thyroid problems and you may be told that the blood lab work has come back "normal". But if thyroid issues go undetected, it can have a serious effect on your over-all health, not just sleep.

BLOOD SUGAR IMBALANCE. If you are sleepy in the middle of the afternoon, or fall asleep when sitting down, the problem may not be your lack of sleep, but your blood sugar. Try eliminating all sugar and bread or cereal products for 3 weeks

PB —

and see if that helps. Eat only a small protein snack before bed, with some good quality fat. Be sure to eat a protein breakfast within an hour after rising. If you are not hungry in the morning and hate eating breakfast, your blood sugar is not on a normal cycle. Your blood sugar should fall at night so that you are ready to eat in the a.m. Eat small, frequent meals with good quality fat and protein at each. Good fats include real butter, unrefined oils, raw coconut oil, raw nut butters, organic dairy products.

TOXICITY/CONGESTION OF LIVER/GALL BLADDER. It is a principle of Chinese medicine that the organs detox at night. If an organ is very congested, that can cause wakefulness. If you wake up between 2 and 4 a.m. and find it difficult to go back to sleep, consider a liver/gall bladder detox. Truthfully, anyone can benefit from a "spring cleaning" for the liver and gall bladder, as the liver is the main detox organ for the blood. Allergies, obesity, cancer, aches and pains, constipation, flatulence, itching skin, skin eruptions like acne and eczema, bad breath, cravings for tobacco, alcohol, drugs and sweets, dry skin, worrying may all be signs of an over-burdened liver.

Dr Christopher's L/GB
detox - Amazon
Barbury bark,
Wild Yam Root,
Cramp Bark,
Fennel seed,
ginger root
Catnip herb
Peppermint leaf

ADRENAL FATIGUE. Fibromyalgia, asthma, allergies, muscular and nervous exhaustion, poor circulation, low blood pressure and anxiety may all be signs of adrenal exhaustion. These symptoms may interfere with restful sleep. See a practitioner who can test and treat adrenals. If you have thyroid issues, suspect adrenal problems as well. The endocrine system works together like an orchestra. You can't expect beautiful music unless all the instruments are being played.

DIGESTION ISSUES. Eat lightly at night after 6 p.m. and take digestive enzymes and probiotics. Most of the patients I see who have a gastric reflux diagnosis actually have a hiatus hernia. Medical doctors don't know how to fix it, but it is a simple adjustment by a Chiropractor or Naturopath. Don't take medication that stops your digestion by lowering your stomach acid like the GURD (gastric reflux) medications do. Most of us need more stomach acid, not less, due to our high sugar, carb and processed food diets. But we need the stomach acid to break down proteins we eat. If indigestion is keeping you up at night, find someone who can actually fix your digestive ability, not mask the symptoms with drugs.

The bottom line is to consider insomnia as a symptom of a deeper problem. The answer is not sleep medication, or psychotropic medication, as the medications themselves are toxic to the organs, have side-effects, are often addictive and may be a short-term crutch that masks or worsens a long-term health problem.

If your medical doctor simply wants to give you medication without identifying the underlying problem, find a practitioner who can really help. Lack of sleep puts tremendous stress on the body. Sleep is a time of healing and repair, and if that is not taking place health can deteriorate rapidly. Life becomes burdensome when the body is exhausted. Treat insomnia as a secondary condition and know that your body is asking for help. Find the real cause of your insomnia and you will be able to correct a health issue that is demanding your attention.

Your body deserves to be rested and refreshed from a good night's sleep. Sweet dreams.

Stress

What is it and how do you get rid of it?

Stress occurs when there is a "burden" or "load" that exceeds the ability or capacity to easily handle. There are 3 types of Stress that affect us.

ENVIRONMENTAL STRESS: coping with an environment that tests our ability to respond to constantly changing stimuli. Traffic, information over-load, juggling time demands of home, family and job.

PHYSIOLOGICAL STRESS: toxins and chemicals bombarding our bodies that tax our body's ability to process the poisons. Artificial fragrances, cleaning products, food additives and chemicals, pharmaceutical drugs, smoking, hormones, petrochemicals cause this type of stress.

EMOTIONAL STRESS: break-ups, divorce, chemical and drug addictions, family strife, work-place relationship challenges.

There is little that can be done about numbers 1 and 3. We live in a fast-paced culture, we have to confront traffic and are bombarded by the media for our attention. Moving to an island and getting rid of our laptops and cell phones might be the only solution.

The ups and downs of relationships is part of what makes us human. The only way to have the joy of love is to also be

Stressed spelled backwards is desserts. Coincidence? I think not!

Author Unknown

open to the pain of loss. Financial stress can bring us closer, or strain us to the breaking point.

The only type of stress that we have immediate control over is number 2. By relieving the toxic burden in our bodies and giving ourselves concentrated nutrients, we can help our organs, glands and cells cope with the assault of chemicals we are exposed to daily.

The good news is that releasing the toxins in the body, and improving the quality of our nutrition, helps us to become emotionally more stable and able to cope with the challenges in our lives.

 Toxins are stored in the fat tissue of our bodies. By releasing fat tissue with HCG, the toxic burden is reduced.

Lose weight, lose the toxins—gain a better quality of life.

What to Check if You Are Not Losing Weight

First of all, check each point on the Debug Checklist. Make the appropriate changes as noted.

The general rule of thumb is that the more weight you need to lose, the stricter you need to be about following the dietary guidelines.

If you have been greatly overweight for many years, your metabolism may need more help to reset.

There are two things I check if there is less weight loss than expected and the person is following the diet as closely as possible: one is thyroid and the other is Gall Bladder.

They are sick that surfeit with too much, as they that starve with nothing.

William Shakespeare

The Gall Bladder is probably most famous for the fact that surgeons remove them all the time simply because they are causing symptoms. This is a little like cutting the wires to the dashboard because the oil light comes on, instead of adding or changing the oil in your car. The Gall Bladder is a vital organ that helps with fat metabolism:

- It neutralizes the acid from the stomach (because bile is very alkaline)

- It breaks down fats so that they can be digested

- It is a natural laxative for the colon

Bile is essential in the digestion of fats. When you eat a meal with fats, the gall bladder releases a LARGE amount of bile to digest the fats. One big problem when a person has gall bladder surgery is that the body has nowhere to store bile until it is needed. Therefore, it just drips continually. And when a large amount is needed to digest a meal with a lot of fat, there is not enough bile available to digest it properly.

Many people, fat and thin, have Gall Bladders that are sluggish. The stuff (bile) that the Gall Bladder squirts out to break up butter, oil and fats in your diet should be thin and slippery. If it becomes thick and sludgy, that can cause symptoms. Toxins from the environment may cause the bile to be sluggish. There is a list of symptoms associated with sluggish Gall Bladder and I see this every day in my practice.

The Gall Bladder may even develop stones, but these are soft, made out of cholesterol (fat) and usually pass easily into the bile duct and out through the intestine. A liver/gall bladder cleanse is a good idea for almost anyone.

Medical doctors remove Gall Bladders when there are stones because they are never taught that there are natural and safe ways to get the stones out.

If you know that you have Gall Bladder symptoms before you start the FAT FIX DIET HCG program it is very important that you take some Gall Bladder support while you are on the drops. You may have some uncomfortable symptoms and it may interfere with speedy weight loss if you don't.

Many people, however, don't realize until they start the program that they have an underlying Gall Bladder issue.

That is why I have included a checklist of symptoms so you can perform a self-test.

Even if a person is missing their Gall Bladder because of surgery, they may still need support for the function of fat metabolism. I recommend that people use Lecithin or Bile salts every day for the rest of their lives. Surgeons will tell you that you don't need your Gall Bladder. But many people have terrible symptoms after surgery, from watery and explosive diarrhea to constipation and weight gain.

The second thing I check for is a low functioning thyroid. The endocrine system is the system that produces hormones or natural chemical messages in the body. The hormones tell the organs like the liver or ovaries or testicles what to do next. There is a wonderful and complex feedback system to the glands and hormones, almost like an orchestra that tries to make beautiful music. The thyroid is the conductor of the orchestra.

One of the most common reasons for infertility in women is a low function thyroid. Although the lab work may place the thyroid hormone in "normal" range, that does not mean the thyroid is functioning as it should. It just means there is no disease and medication is not indicated. But many symptoms are relieved when the thyroid gland is supported with natural supplements, and weight loss is often enhanced. A well-functioning thyroid is also protection against breast cancer.

once start, have to continue.

I have included here a list of thyroid and also adrenal symptoms so you can perform a self-test on the function of these vital glands. The adrenals also may contribute to weight issues as adrenal hormones may communicate with fat cells and contribute to stubborn belly fat being difficult to melt down.

We now know that fat cells can take on a life of their own and interact with the rest of the body like an organ! But this happens in an undesirable way most often when the rest of the hormonal system is out of balance, such as after menopause, andropause (male equivalent of menopause), or when insulin levels are out of balance and blood sugar is unregulated.

5000 years of us Chinese medicine teaches us that optimal health is balanced function of each system in the body.

Debug Checklist

Use this list if you are not losing weight. This list includes all the major points that must be followed. It also suggests changes in the diet that might break a stall, a plateau or lack of substantial weight loss.

Are you eating any foods that are not listed as allowed foods?	Examples would be lamb, pork, processed or luncheon meats, tropical fruits like mango, papaya, banana or pineapple, watermelon, artificial sweeteners, artificial flavorings, processed foods, grains, cereals, breads (other than the allowed bread sticks or melba toast), sugars such as honey, agave, or brown sugar.
Are you eating too late at night?	Don't eat past 8 p.m.
Are you staying up too late?	The body's natural rhythm may be interrupted by staying up past midnight. Night time sleep is used by the body to heal, repair, and recharge. Studies show that animals will gain weight.
Are you getting too little sleep?	Most people do best on 7-9 hours of sleep. On the Fat Fix Diet program it is best to get plenty of rest so that the body has a chance to do the work of melting down the excess fat and processing toxins that are released from the fat cells.

Are you over-exerting through exercise or job demands?	Only mild to moderate physical activity is suggested. If you put too great a demand on the body, appetite may increase and the hormone balance upset. You might need to divide up your protein more, or even increase your protein slightly if you have a physically demanding job, or must exercise hard.
Are you using any artificial sweeteners or chewing gum?	Only Stevia is allowed as a sweetener. Stevia gum is allowed.
Have you been losing steadily for 10-14 days and suddenly not losing for 2-3 days?	This seems to be a normal pattern. Have an apple day or wait it out. *or a steak / Protein day*
Are you drinking too much water? *Sport Drink*	Cut your water back to 2 quarts if you have been drinking more. Try adding a potassium supplement or a pinch of sea salt to water with juice of half lemon and some Stevia for a natural sports drink.
Are you avoiding salt?	Salt is necessary for the cells to let go of waste products. If you are used to eating processed foods, and now you switched to whole foods and are not using salt, you may need to add a little sea salt to your diet. The human body, like all mammals, requires some salt, so salt is not a bad thing and will not contribute to high blood pressure unless used to excess.
Are you constipated? *Yogi Detox Tea + Fiber Tabs*	Check Gall Bladder information for advice. The intestine gets a signal from the release of bile from the gall bladder that it may be missing on the no-fat diet. You may need some gall bladder support or try taking a magnesium supplement or herbal tea like Smooth Move.

Vegetables?	Eat a plate of steamed vegetables, sticking to the allowed list. Only eat 1 type of vegetable at a time if you are stuck and trying to budge the weight.
Salads?	Eat a big, fresh organic salad with lots of dark leafy greens.
Is it close to your period?	Some women seem to stop losing or even gain for a couple of days around the start of their period. Often the weight then drops after the first two days.
Are you using oil-based lotions or creams on face or body?	Some people seem to be able to use these without it stopping their weight loss. Others do well if they are strict. See list of oil-free skin products for suggestions.
Weight Plateau?	Check the scale and see if the weight that you are stalled at is a weight where you hit a plateau before. The body seems to be a creature of habit. Try going to bed earlier, walking a bit more, changing your food from meat to fish, or shaking up your habits a bit to see if you can break the plateau. You may also take a few more drops, from 15 instead of 12, or add another dose of drops at bedtime to see if that helps.
Are you using any processed foods?	Check ingredients on any packaged foods you are using. There are many words for sugar (see list) and you should be avoiding all chemicals as they may cause water retention and/or toxicity.

Are you eating out at a lot because of work or travel?

Understand that you may lose at a slower rate, but you can still lose. Restaurant food may not be the same quality you would get at home, and there may be chemicals and fats, no matter how much you ask for plain food. A green salad and plain chicken breast with lemon squeezed on is a good lunch or dinner choice.

opt > *dressing on side*

Are you watching your protein serving size?

Don't eat more protein at one time than is suggested. Eat slowly and chew food well—it takes a few minutes for the body to get the signals. You may split your protein portion and save for a snack if you need to eat more frequently.

or lunch next day

Sluggish Gall Bladder

This may have contributed to your weight difficulties in the first place. The Gall Bladder has everything to do with fat metabolism. On the no-fat diet, the Gall Bladder may be even more sluggish. Take the self-test for Gall Bladder and use the recommended supplements. You may wish to stay on these supplements after your Fat Fix Diet program and into the Maintenance and Forever After phases. Doctors remove the Gall Bladder like it was a hang-nail, but it is a vital organ and can be helped, without surgery, even if there are gall stones.

Thyroid or Adrenal?

Take the self-test for Thyroid and Adrenal. If you have had your thyroid checked with blood work and the lab results came back in the "normal" range, you may still have a thyroid that is not functioning at the optimal level. You can take some natural thyroid support if you have the symptoms listed and assist your thyroid to work better. This is good for your health and may help you to lose weight. This approach is called "Functional Medicine".

Dizziness	This may mean that your blood sugar has dropped too low. Try adding Cinnamon to your eating plan. Use it liberally on fruit, such as baked apples. May also take in a supplement form.
Dizziness and weakness	Try adding more sea salt to your food, especially in warm and humid weather. If you are on blood pressure medication you should have your blood pressure monitored closely. The Fat Fix program may cause your blood pressure to drop and the medication may no longer be needed.
Muscle and Leg Cramps	Take Magnesium supplements, especially at night before bedtime, if night cramps are a problem. Be sure you are drinking enough water. You may also need some potassium, if you are urinating frequently or you live in a hot or humid climate.

If you experience headaches the first few days of the program, it is a symptom that you may need some liver/gall bladder support. Headaches do not happen to very many and they do not last.

Secret Plateau Buster

Don't use this tip often; only if you don't lose for 3-4 days and you have been following the FAT FIX DIET Program very strictly. Check all the points of the Debug Checklist first.

If you feel you are genuinely stuck, eat a small amount of fat at bedtime. Eat a little cheese on a cracker (1 oz.,) eat a teaspoon or two of butter, or take a teaspoon or two of olive oil on some veggies or crackers. A teaspoon of half and half or cream may also be used. Choose one of these fats that you enjoy and use it for one night.

In other words, break the diet a bit. Your body may need to get some fat into the system again to trigger further release of fat from the cells.

The Homeopathic HCG is all about "tweaking". Homeopathy seems to act as a little trigger or switch in the body to help it do something it is trying to do anyway. Because it "tweaks", instead of a punch you get a little love-tap. This makes it pretty safe and a lot of fun to use.

Thyroid Symptoms

Place a check mark next to symptoms that you experience frequently.

☑ Symptom	☑ Symptom
☑ Hair Loss	☐ Dry, breaking brittle hair
☑ Cold body temperature	☐ Panic Attacks
☐ Nervous Weight Gain	☑ Can't lose weight *(1000-1200 cal or less)*
☑ Low libido (pronounced)	☐ Irritability
☐ Anxiety or nervousness	☐ Sleep Disturbances
☐ Fatigue	☐ Feeling "Burned Out"
☑ Bone, muscle, strength loss *- Exercise*	☐ Unusual sweating
☐ Difficulty falling asleep	☑ Thinning papery skin
☐ Sad or depressed without cause	☐ Decreased concentration
☐ Short attention span	☐ Dry, breaking, brittle nails
☐ Aches and Pains systemically	☑ (Goiter)
☐ Tremors in fingers	☑ Memory lapses *Some*
☑ High cholesterol	☐ Mood changes-Mood swings
☐ Low blood pressure	☐ Slow pulse rate
☐ Difficulty swallowing	☐ Weight gain
☐ Depressed or moody	☑ Constipated
☐ Hair loss	☐ Feeling cold when others don't
☐ Low sex drive	☐ Forgetfulness

☑ Symptom	☑ Symptom
☐ Gall stones or sluggish gall bladder	☐ Slower heartbeat
☐ Muscle cramps	☐ Muscle weakness
☐ Constipation	☐ Poor circulation
☐ Weight Loss (Rapid)	☑ Cold hands and feet
☐ Erratic behavior	☐ Heart Palpitations
☐ Bulging or protruding eyes	☐ Feeling hot most of the time
☐ Infertility	☐ Insomnia
☐ Vertical ridges on fingernails	☐ Rapid heartbeat
☐ Inability to focus or concentrate	☐ Forgetful
☐ Edema with puffy face & eyes	☐ Decreased sweating
☐ Frequently tired	☑ Dry skin or hair; brittle nails
☐ Infertility or recurrent miscarriage	☐ Painful or erratic periods
☐ Throat pain	☐ Hypertension
☐ Suicidal tendencies	

Tally your score. ☐ 12 ☐

A score of 4 or more symptoms indicates low function of the thyroid. See the Supplements section for recommended Thyroid supplements.

Adrenal Symptoms

Place a check by symptoms that you experience frequently.

☑ Symptom	☑ Symptom
☐ Fatigue	☐ Bone loss
☐ Allergies	☑ Weight gain–waist
☐ Nervous Weight Gain	☐ Sleep disturbance
☐ Stress	☐ Elevated triglycerides
☐ Breast cancer	☐ Arthritis
☐ Anxious feeling in chest in a.m.	☐ Nervous
☐ Depression	☐ Irritability
☐ Decreased concentration	☐ Stress
☑ Low libido *Th ?*	☐ Low immunity
☐ Headaches	☐ Masculine Tendencies (female)
☐ Panic	☐ Anxiety
☐ Dizziness	☐ Hot Flashes
☑ Craving sugar	☐ Chemical sensitivity
☐ Insomnia	☐ Heart Palpitations
☐ Irritable	☐ Aches and Pains
☐ Headaches	☑ Cold body Temperature *thyroid ?*
☐ Chronic Fatigue	☐ Respiratory disorders
☐ Arthritis	

Tally your score. ☐ 4 ☐ *– thyroid 2 ?*

If you have a score of 5 or more, see "Supplements for Success" on page 84 for recommended Adrenal supplements to add to your program.

Gall Bladder Symptoms

Place a check next to symptoms you experience frequently.

☑ Symptom	☑ Symptom
☐ Pain/tenderness right shoulder blade or between shoulder blades	☑ Dry skin
☑ Constipation-needs laxatives *(Fiber Tabs)*	☐ Wakes during night with anxiety and worries
☐ Burning anus	☐ Difficulty digesting fatty foods
☑ Crave sweets	☑ Hair falling out
☐ History of gall stones	☑ Bloating
☐ Headaches before period	☐ Frequent or severe *grains* stomach upset
☐ History of morning sickness	☑ High cholesterol
☐ Burning feet	☑ Intolerance for milk products *phlegm*
☐ Light colored stool	☐ Nightmares
☐ Migraines	☐ Queasiness
☐ Difficulty losing weight	

Tally your score. ☐ 7

If you have a score of 2 or more, see the Supplements section for gall bladder support.

Almost anyone can use Gall Bladder support on the FAT FIX DIET program because of the low fat eating plan. If you have had Gall Bladder surgery, you should use Gall Bladder support every day, as the function of the gall bladder (fat handling) still exists.

Dear God,
All I ask for in 2011 is a big fat bank account and a slim body. Please don't mix them up like you did last year.
Amen !!! ;'j-

If you have headaches or constipation after starting the program, add Gall Bladder support. The program will not cause a problem, but it may reveal an underlying issue that can be corrected, improving your health and fat metabolism while you lose weight.

Supplements for Success

Here is what to take if your score shows you need extra supplements:

Thyroid

There are supplements that will help the thyroid to function better, or assist your thyroid medication to work better for you. If you are currently on thyroid medication, but your score showed you need additional help, supplements may give you the balance your body needs. Not only will uncomfortable symptoms disappear, but your body will be much healthier. The hormonal system works together like an orchestra, and the thyroid is the orchestra leader.

I like *Thytrophin PMG* from Standard Process Supplements. Many people will also benefit from iodine supplementation. There are many toxins that interfere with iodine receptors in the body, even if you have enough iodine in your diet, and few of us eat enough iodine rich foods.

For iodine supplementation I like Lugol's liquid iodine, or *Iodomere* from Standard Process. Start with 2 drops Lugol's and increase 1 drop per week for 6 weeks, then stay at that dosage for several months. May take 1–2 Iodomere per day. Sufficient iodine is not only beneficial for thyroid, but helps the immune system and is associated with low cancer risk for breast and prostate cancer.

Adrenals

Coffee, sugar, stress, late nights—all a recipe for adrenal exhaustion. If your score indicates weak adrenals, you will feel much more energy and stability from taking supplements.

The adrenal glands store the most Vitamin C in the body. But try to get whole food sources of C, such as strawberries and oranges. Supplements include *Cataplex C* from Standard Process, as well as *Drenamin*. Eluthero is a calming herb for the adrenals, while licorice extract is a more stimulating herb.

Gall Bladder

Because of the extremely low fat eating plan, during the use of the Magic Drops HCG, almost anyone can use gall bladder support. The gall bladder normally scoops up bile that was produced by the liver. Bile is stored in the gall bladder and released when you eat any kind of fat, like salad dressing or cheese. The bile acts as an emulsifier to break down fat into small particles that are absorbed and use for energy in the body.

When the bile gets too thick, like heavy cream, the gall bladder is sluggish and the bile does not flow out into the bile duct to break up the fat. Eventually gallstones are formed. Fortunately gallstones are soft like cooked peas, and they can be flushed out with a gall bladder cleanse. A gall bladder flush is not a bad idea for anyone to do. See recipe at the end of this section. (Check with your physician before hand if you are being treated for any medical condition.)

Another safe way to make sure that your gall bladder is "happy" during the FAT FIX DIET program is to use gall bladder supplements. I recommend *AF Betafood* or *Betafood* from Standard Process. These are whole food supplements made from beet extract that thins the bile and allows the bile to flow easily into the bile duct to emulsify dietary fat.

If you know or suspect that you have gallstones, add *Disodium Phosphate* from Standard Process. Follow directions on the box. Please note that Disodium Phosphate is a high salt product, in case your physician has you on sodium restriction.

Even if you have had your gall bladder removed, the function of the gall bladder to break down fat is still there. You should take Lecithin every day after gall bladder surgery.

More About Supplements

Since you can eat unlimited quantities of vegetables on the eating plan, you may find that you are getting more nutrition than before. If you want to give yourself more of a boost, or if you have had allergies or immune issues, you can use a multivitamin. Again, your body will benefit the most from food source supplements. *Catalyn*, from Standard Process was the original multivitamin developed in 1929 and is still the top choice. *Cataplex B* is a natural B complex. *Enzycore* and *Multizyme* are digestive enzymes that will help you get all the nutrition from the food you are eating, as well as help with allergies and inflammation. *Zypan* is excellent for protein digestion.

Candida and Intestinal Health

Many of us have had far too many antibiotics, which destroy the "good" bugs as well as the disease causing pathogens. The intestine is dependent on the good bugs to help us digest food and makes vitamins, as well as being a major part of our immune system. Probiotics can be very helpful during the FAT FIX DIET program, to help clean up the gut while the burden of white flour and white sugar is lifted. If gas and bloating has been a problem, try *Zymex* or *Zymex II* from Standard Process. They will help break down undigested carbohydrate that feeds candida. *Lact Enz* is excellent if you have been eating a lot of dairy. It is not the number of different colonies that makes a difference with probiotics. There is no evidence that all the different kinds of organisms are able to actually seed in our gut. Acidophilus is still the most important colony to replace.

The Thyroid, Iodine and Weight Loss

The thyroid gland is a major factor in metabolic rate, which means how your body breaks down and utilizes the food you eat. You may know people who seem to be able to eat anything and never gain weight. Others may feel they just look at a cookie and gain a pound or two. – me !

> If you really want to be depressed, weigh yourself in grams.
> **Jason Love**

The thyroid is like the orchestra leader for your glandular/endocrine system. Your hormones tell the organs and other glands what to do. This creates a network of communication. When all the glands are working well, they will create harmony and music in the body. So, keeping the thyroid gland functioning well is one of the keys to health, longevity and weight stability.

The thyroid must have iodine in order to make thyroid hormones. Medical doctors don't tell you this. They also don't tell you that lab work for thyroid measures disease, not wellness. You may be told that your thyroid is "normal" even when you are tired, depressed and over-weight. What you are really being told is that you do not have thyroid disease that requires medication.

If you want to know how well your thyroid is functioning, check the list of thyroid symptoms and see how you score. Natural nutritional thyroid supplements do not contain hormones and are not drugs, so they can be used safely.

You may also consider iodine supplementation, and eating seaweed, which is the best source of iodine. I like Lugol's iodine or Iodomere. Iodized salt may not be enough, nor is it the best form of iodine for the body to utilize.

> "Iodine is necessary for the thyroid gland's proper performance of its work. All the blood in the body passes through the thyroid gland every 17 minutes. Because the cells making up this gland have an affinity for iodine, during this 17-minute passage the gland's secretion of iodine kills weak germs that may have gained entry into the blood through an injury to the skin, the lining of nose or throat, or through absorption of food from the digestive tract. Strong, virulent germs are rendered weaker during their passage through the thyroid gland. With each 17 minutes that rolls around they are made still weaker until finally they are killed if the gland has its normal supply of iodine. If it does not, it cannot kill harmful germs circulating in the blood as Nature intended it should."
>
> Dr. D.C. Jarvis
> Vermont Country Medicine

I have seen dramatic improvements in mental outlook and physical health when the thyroid is helped. Fatigue disappears and weight is easier to lose. If you have struggled with overweight for a long time, do consider supporting your thyroid and supplementing with iodine.

No one is allergic to iodine, by the way. That would be like saying someone was allergic to calcium. Iodine is a mineral that is vital for human health. Cretinism is a medical term for someone who is low IQ due to iodine deficiency. It is always a good idea to start iodine supplementation very slowly, as it can turn on a detox effect that may be confused for allergy. Start Lugol's iodine with just 2 drops per day *dose* and increase slowly to 6 drops and maintain that for a few months. If you feel any detox effect, simply back down on the amount. I rarely see a problem when used this way. Start with 1 Iodomere per day for the first week. You may increase to 3-4 Iodomere over the next 3 weeks and maintain that dose for a few months.

Ovarian cysts, breast cancer and prostate cancer may be prevented by supplementing with iodine, according to Dr. David Brownstein. See his blog at www.drbrownstein.com

Constipation

The change in eating pattern may cause constipation, particularly in those already prone to be sluggish normally. Be sure to drink enough water, but don't over-do it. One half gallon is enough for most people. You can try Smooth Move tea, or there are many herbal preparations that work, but look for something gentle. Try eating a big plate of steamed veggies for a day or two. Applesauce or eating a couple of apples a day is helpful for some. Sedona Labs makes a probiotic called I Flora which helps many people to be more regular.

Fiber
Water
Tea
Veg
Apples
Probiotic

Medications and Medical Conditions

Of course, anyone who is on a medication or being treated for a medical condition should consult his or her physician before starting a new diet or treatment.

Generally, homeopathy does not interfere or interact with any medications. The homeopathic HCG is not hormone replacement and there is no discernible HCG hormone in the drops, as is true of all homeopathic preparations. It is the "imprint" of the substance that makes the homeopathic remedy effective. This also makes homeopathy very safe.

Teens

Teenagers can use the program successfully. Take into consideration their life-style. If they are involved in heavy sports programs it would be better to wait until they are between sports. They may need more protein and food in general, due to their growing bodies. However, with some minor adjustments, teens will slim down and often acne will disappear. A teen who is eating junk food and drinking soda will benefit enormously from eating according to this plan. And they may realize for themselves that they feel better eating whole foods. If acne is a problem, coffee should be eliminated, also, as well as any other caffeinated drinks.

Some medications may have to be adjusted while on the program. Blood pressure medication, cholesterol medication and diabetes medication may all need to be reduced. If you are on these medications, please note that you will need to consult your physician and monitor yourself carefully. This eating plan is an ideal way to reduce the need for medications and correct the underlying metabolic imbalances that created the need for them in the first place.

Thyroid Medication

If you are on thyroid medication or other hormone replacement, you may be hungrier on the diet and need extra food or an extra dose of drops every day. The diet

90

will be helpful for hormone imbalances. You may want to take some extra support for the endocrine system as listed in the section on Supplements. Iodine supplementation is usually indicated for anyone who has a thyroid issue or sluggish metabolism.

Menstrual Cycle

Menstrual pain and PMS may be greatly benefited by this program. Often cramps improve greatly when wheat is eliminated from the diet. A woman will often gain a couple of pounds if she has her period while on the diet. This weight gain is usually temporary.

Acid Blockers and Gastric Reflux

Very few people have too much stomach acid. The reason they have stomach distress is because they have too little! Although acid blockers provide symptomatic relief, reducing acid production affects digestion. The only way to get vital nutrients to the cells that need them is through the process of complete digestion. You have 46 trillion cells in your body and each one is a unique living organism that needs fuel and building blocks to function and create new healthy cells. New cells are made when existing cells divide. So, you might say that your body is "pregnant" all the time, because a billion new cells are made every hour. The food you eat provides the building material for the new cells. So, when the choice is donuts and French fries, or broccoli and spinach, guess how your cells would vote.

I am a nutritional overachiever.

Author Unknown

If digestion is interrupted and the food particles are too large when they hit the intestine, the nutrients cannot be absorbed through the intestinal walls into the blood for transport to the cells.

Chew more !

91

If you are on acid blockers, at least add in some digestive enzymes to give a helping hand. Everyone can use extra digestive enzymes. If you have difficulty digesting meat, the answer is to improve your digestion. Meat has been demonized, but humans have survived on meat for thousands of years and it is not true that meat causes cancer. There was very little cancer before the twentieth century, and cancer rates have soared since the introduction of hydrogenated fats (shortening and margarine), processed white flours and grains and heavy use of white sugar and high-fructose corn syrup, not to mention all the chemicals from industry and agriculture. Red meat is a real, whole food and it is natural for our bodies to have meat in the diet.

Regardless of what kind of protein you eat, only people who actually have ulcers or some other rare issue with the stomach and esophagus need acid blockers. Find a practitioner who can help you get your digestion fixed so it is functioning well, as it is key to health and longevity.

This eating program will take some of the burden off digestion, so you may have less need for gastric reflux medication.

Psychiatric Medication and Mood Enhancers

The homeopathic HCG program usually enhances feelings of well being because of the anti-inflammatory aspect of the eating plan. Many people are affected badly by eating certain kinds of foods. Taking the diet back to the basics of protein, fruits and vegetables takes a burden off the organs and glands, and often a person will feel more cheerful and positive as a result. The drops themselves will not affect medication. It is the combination of the drops and way of eating that helps people to feel better. For more information on the dangers and side-effects of psychiatric medication, please visit www.cchr.org.

Sleep

Improved sleep is commonly reported. You may want to try taking one dose of the drops in the evening. The HCG drops will help to balance blood sugar, which may improve sleep. Many people have reported that they were able to stop using sleep medications while on the FAT FIX DIET and no longer need chemical assistance for sleep.

Over The Counter Medications

It is best to avoid any over the counter medications as much as possible while on the program. Many people have reduces pain and head aches, so the need for pain relievers is often reduced.

Some people do experience a mild headache the first day or few days on the program. When you break down fat tissue, there may be a release of toxins that were "fat-loving" and stored in the fat. Gall bladder support supplements may help. See section on supplements on gall bladder symptoms.

More Supplement Options

I recommend Standard Process supplements because I have used them in my practice for twenty years, with outstanding results. Standard Process sells only through health practitioners, and for a reason. Doctors and nutritionists who use Standard Process supplements have been through hours of training to learn how to use them effectively.

You may contact the doctors on the Distributor page to order Standard Process supplements, or contact the company at www.standardprocess.com for the name of a practitioner near you.

Please do not order Standard Process supplements online. The company has a very strict company policy about selling the products online and anyone who is selling them directly from a website is doing so disreputably. If you have a health practitioner who uses another line of supplements, they will be able to help you find substitute products.

Lugol's iodine may be ordered through my office at 818 729 9149, or online at Jcrows.com/iodine.

Xymogen makes some excellent products. If you are using an estrogen hormone product, prescription or bio-identical, I recommend *DIM* from Xymogen. It is also helpful for men with prostate problems, or those who wish to avoid developing prostate issues. DIM is an extract of cruciferous vegetables. This group of vegetables, kale, broccoli, cabbage and brussels sprouts, are rich in sulfur, which are vital for liver detoxification. Xymogen also makes supplements for thyroid and gall bladder/liver support.

Gall Bladder Cleanse/Stone Flush

Do this cleanse before you start the FAT FIX DIET program. Prepare for the cleanse by taking 12 *AF Betafood* or 10 *Betafood* from Standard Process daily for 2 weeks. Or you may drink 1-2 glasses of organic apple juice for two weeks. This will soften the stones so that they will come out easily during the flush.

Ingredients:

> 1/2 Cup(= 1.25 dl) Olive Oil Extra Virgin
>
> 2 grapefruits

Juice of 4 fresh organic lemons

4 tablespoons of Epsom Salts = $MgSO_4$ = Magnesium Sulfate

or

Disodium Phosphate Capsules

3 cups water (=750 dl)

Choose a time to do the flush when you have a couple of days when you can relax and stay close to a bathroom. Eat a normal breakfast and a light lunch.

Two hours after lunch, take a dose of Epsom Salts, 1-2 TBLS in a glass of warm water (bigger body, more Epsom Salts). May use 10 capsules of Disodium Phosphate instead.

For dinner have another dose of Epsom Salts or 10 Disodium Phosphate and eat 2 grapefruit only.

At bedtime, drink ½ cup extra virgin olive oil, mixed with the fresh lemon juice. Sipping through a straw may help it go down easier.

Go to bed and lie on right side.

In morning take another dose of Epsom Salts or Disodium Phosphate. Two hours later, eat a light breakfast.

Watch for stones in stool. Often they look like greenish-brown lumps.

This cleanse may be repeated 2-3 times, waiting at least 2 weeks between flushes.

If you have any medical conditions, check with your physician before doing this cleanse/flush. Medical doctors do not realize that gallbladder stones release and do not require surgery unless the gallbladder itself is badly diseased.

Many people experience a drastic reduction in symptoms after one or more gallbladder cleanses. These symptoms include acne, fatigue, insomnia, constipation, indigestion, hot flashes and back pain.

Note: If you are on a salt restricted diet, choose the Epsom Salts.

Metabolism-What Is It?

Metabolism is the word we use for the chemical and physical processes of ingesting foodstuff, breaking it down into basic parts, and using those basic parts for production of energy (fuel for activity) and the repair and formation of cells and other body components.

Imagine that you decide to build a house entirely of wood. You go to the forest and cut down trees. You cut some of the wood into thick lengths and lay out the shape of the house. Some of the wood is cut into thin planks for walls. Pegs are fashioned to hold the walls in place. Flooring is cut, doors made to size, windows set. Furniture is custom made and built in. Decorative pieces are carved for the shutters and roof. Each wooden piece is made to order for this house. When it is finished, the house is unique and as strong as you are precise about how it all fits together.

This is like metabolism. Big things are broken down into smaller pieces and then re-fashioned as needed to create something new and unique.

An example would be eating meat, fish or chicken (protein) and breaking down the protein into amino acids. There are eight amino acids that are called "essential" because humans can't make them, but must acquire them from food. Plants do contain proteins, but they do not contain the eight essential amino acids. Plants must be combined to form complete

No diet will remove all the fat from your body because the brain is entirely fat. Without a brain, you might look good, but all you could do is run for public office.

George Bernard Shaw

97

proteins. Beans and rice are used together in many cuisines to form more complete proteins. Only meats, poultry, fish, eggs and dairy products contain all essential amino acids.

How can you increase your metabolism? Eat whole, natural unprocessed foods. The body can break down and utilize foods it recognizes. Our bodies are natural ecosystems. The friendly bacteria in our guts help breakdown our foods, and produce vitamins we cannot make ourselves. To keep this gut colony healthy, unrefined foods are vital, as well as naturally fermented foods such as kefir, yogurt, raw cheese, sauerkraut, and tempeh (fermented soy).

White flour, white sugar, processed fats, chemicals and synthetic Frankenstein foods cannot be utilized for fuel or cellular function. They cause inflammation clog our digestive tract. Frankenstein foods create Frankenstein bodies, since food contains the building blocks for making new cells.

When it comes to fats, just consult Mother Nature. Real butter, fish oils, virgin vegetable oils, raw nuts, raw (unpasteurized/heat-treated) dairy products and meats have been consumed by humans for all of recorded history. Heart disease was virtually unknown before 1900. Margarine was invented in the late 1880s. Heat and chemically processed oils were added in the effort to find cheap fats with long shelf lives.

Let's go back to your wooden house. Now imagine only half-emptying the waste-baskets and kitchen trash. Pile up old newspapers and dirty rags. Leave dirty dishes and the remains of your meals. How long before rodents, bacteria and insects would find a feast? Eventually the garbage would spill out into the yard and the smell would announce your lack of housekeeping to the neighborhood.

If you clog up the body with waste it cannot breakdown and eliminate, parasitic bugs and yeast organisms start to thrive.

Eat Real

Whatever you decide to eat, choose "live" unprocessed food that has a very short shelf life and your body will get the metabolic boost it needs to help you stay slim and healthy.

Ever wonder how cows get so big when their native diet is grass? Cows are "ruminants" which means they have multiple stomachs, instead of just one like humans. Humans have a hundred trillion good "bugs" in their gut, but cows have a hundred times that many. These helpful bacteria break down cellulose into carbohydrates, proteins and fats, as well as vitamins and minerals, that cows use to make their big bodies. Cows must eat 10 hours a day in order to ingest enough calories.

Adult African elephants, also herbivores, eat 220-440 lbs of vegetation per day. A herbivore is an animal that eats only plants in the wild. Gorillas are herbivores who become very strong on a diet of fruits, leaves and tree bark. Adult males eat about 50 lbs of food per day.

Notice that herbivores must eat huge quantities of food and spend most of their waking hours foraging for food!

Frankenstein Foods and Additives To Avoid

Hydrogenated fats such as margarine and shortening. Hydrogenation extends shelf life but changes the chemical structure of the fat to something the human body has never had to process before. Saturated fats are not a health risk, but <u>trans-fats</u> from hydrogenation or high heat frying are a risk. <u>Coconut oil</u> may be solid, depending the temperature of the room, but it is not an hydrogenated fat and <u>has many health benefi</u>ts, including some promise as a treatment for Alzheimer's.

Liquid Vegetable Oils that have been heat and chemical processed. This would include all oils on the grocery store shelf that are not labeled "Unrefined", "Raw" or "Virgin, cold pressed".

Artificial Sweeteners such as aspartame, sucralose and saccharine. Brand names are Nutrasweet, Sweet and Low and Splenda. Sucralose (Splenda) is sugar chemically bonded with chlorine so that it tastes sweet but does not break down in the body but passes through the intestine.

High Fructose Corn Syrup. This is a manufactured (laboratory-made) sugar created from corn starch. A combination of glucose and fructose, it is much sweeter than glucose, and mixes well with liquids such as sodas, and is

All people are made alike – of bones and flesh and dinner. — Only the dinners are different.

Gertrude Louise Cheney

cheaper than cane or beet sugar. This is good news for soda manufacturers, but bad news for humans. Rats fed liquids with HFCS added become obese. It is hard to make a rat get fat, but HFCS and MSG will do it.

MSG, Autolyzed Yeast, Flavor Enhancers. Monosodium Glutamate exists naturally in seaweed and was used by the Japanese as a flavor booster. But the synthetic, laboratory-made MSG has been used to cause obesity in laboratory mice and rats, and has been linked to brain lesions. It may also cause uncomfortable symptoms such as headache, numbness and tingling.

Food colorings and flavorings. These chemicals have been linked to hyperactivity in children and may contribute to food addictions and allergies. No laboratory can match the taste of a real, ripe strawberry, but that does not stop food companies from making cheap imitations.

Processed, packaged foods. Check the label. If you see words with several syllables that you can't pronounce and you don't know what they are, chances are your body can't process the additive and anything the body can't process acts like a poison. Refined flour and white sugar are the least of the health risks for many processed foods.

Eat Real, Be Real.

Water vs. Coke

Water

1. 75% of Americans are chronically dehydrated. (Likely applies to half the world population)

2. In 37% of Americans, the thirst mechanism is so weak that it is mistaken for hunger.

3. Even MILD dehydration will slow down one's metabolism as much as 3%.

> Gluttony is not a secret vice.
>
> **Orson Welles**

4. One glass of water will shut down midnight hunger pangs for almost 100% of the dieters studied in a University of Washington study.

5. Lack of water is the #1 trigger of daytime fatigue.

6. Preliminary research indicates that 8-10 glasses of water a day could significantly ease back and joint pain for up to 80% of sufferers.

7. A mere 2% drop in body water can trigger fuzzy short-term memory loss, trouble with basic math, and difficulty focusing on the computer screen or on a printed page.

8. Drinking 5 glasses of water daily decreases the risk of colon cancer by 45%, plus it can slash the risk of breast cancer by 79%, and one is 50% less likely to develop bladder cancer.

Are you drinking the amount of water you should drink every day?

 Cola

1. Cola is very acidic with a pH of 2.525. Battery acid has a pH of 1.0. Pure water at room temperature has a pH of 7.0.

2. Teeth immersed in colas and other soft drinks lost 5% of the weight of the enamel.

3. To remove rust spots from chrome car bumpers:

4. Rub the bumper with a rumpled-up piece of aluminum foil dipped in cola.

5. To clean corrosion from car battery terminals: Pour a can of cola over the terminals to bubble away the corrosion.

6. To loosen a rusted bolt: Apply a cloth soaked in cola to the rusted bolt for several minutes.

7. To bake a moist ham: Empty a can of cola into the baking pan, wrap the ham in aluminum foil, and bake.

8. Thirty minutes before ham is finished, remove the foil, allowing the drippings to mix with the Coke for a sumptuous brown gravy.

9. To remove grease from clothes: Empty a can of cola into the load of greasy clothes, add detergent, and run through a regular cycle. The cola will help loosen grease stains. It will also clean road haze from your windshield.

FOR YOUR INFORMATION:

The active ingredient in cola is phosphoric acid.

It will dissolve a nail in about four days. Phosphoric acid also leaches calcium from bones and is a major contributor to the rising increase of osteoporosis.

 To carry coke syrup (the concentrate) the commercial trucks must use a Hazardous Material sign.

Starring!! Your Body!

Most people know more about their favorite sports team or the latest celebrity news than they do about how their own bodies work.

The word "doctor" comes from the Latin "docere", which means to teach. But how many doctors have the time or inclination to teach us what we need to know to keep our body healthy?

Here are some astounding facts about your body:

> Your body is the baggage you must carry through life. The more excess the baggage, the shorter the trip.
>
> **Arnold H. Glasgow**

- There are approximately 60 to 100 trillion cells in the adult body.

- Every hour approximately 2 billion cells must be replaced.

- Where do dead cells go? To the kidney, to be excreted.

- A human body has 60,000 miles of blood vessels.

- 3 million red blood cells are made in the human body every second.

- One million white blood cells are made every second.

- The heart pumps about 2,000 gallons of blood through those vessels every day.

- The average heart beats 100,000 times per day.

- The average human heart will beat 3,000 million times in its lifetime and pump 48 million gallons of blood.

- There are 30 trillion blood cells in the human body.

- There are about 6 quarts of blood in the adult body. The blood circulates through the body three times every minute.

- The lungs contain 300 billion capillaries.

- 400 gallons of blood are pumped (and filtered) through the kidneys every day.

- Each red blood cell lives an average of 120 days. The spleen is a recycling plant for red blood cells.

- The human heart creates enough pressure to squirt blood 30 feet.

- The human body is comprised of about 75% water.

- The lining of the digestive system is shed every 3 days.

- The average surface of the human intestine is 656 square feet.

- The brain can function at a rate of over 100,000 chemical reactions per second.

- The heart is the strongest muscle. There are 650 muscles in the body.

- It takes 30 muscles to smile and 200 muscles to take one step.

- The eye blinks over 10,000,000 a year.

- Your skin weighs twice as much as your brain .

- The skin is about 1/20 of an inch thick.

- Every square inch of the skin contains about 19,000,000 skin cells.

- There are 450 hairs in the average eyebrow.

- Each human tooth has about 55 canals in it.

- The surface of the human skin is 25 square feet.

- There are 45 miles of nerves in the human skin.

- You lose enough dead skin in your lifetime to fill 8 five pound flour bags. That is 600,000 cells of skin every hour!

- The human nose can remember 50,000 different scents.

- The tongue has 9,000 taste buds.

- During a 24-hour period, the average human will breathe 23,040 times.

- Adults lungs have over 600 million tiny air sacs called alveoli.

- 20% of the oxygen we breathe goes to the brain.

- The air from a human sneeze can travel at *(Cover)* speeds of 100 miles per hour or more.

- The body contains over 1,600 types of protein, each made of a different combination of 20-22 amino acids.

- In a lifetime, the average person produces about 25,000 quarts of saliva — enough to fill two swimming pools!

- The small intestine is 22 feet long.

- Stomach acid (hydrochloric acid) is strong enough to corrode steel, but the stomach protects itself by making a new mucosa lining every three to four days.

- The liver performs 500 functions in the body, including detoxifying chemicals and other toxins that enter through the mouth or nose.

- Pound for pound a human baby is as strong as an ox.

- A pair of feet have 500,000 sweat glands and can produce more than a pint of sweat a day.

- There are 54 bones in each hand and wrist.

- The hardest substance in the human body is tooth enamel.

- The femur (thigh bone) is the strongest and longest bone in the body, and the bone itself is harder than concrete, but the femur is hollow so that it is light enough to be lifted.

- The average adolescent girl has approximately 34,000 egg follicles in the ovaries.

- The smallest cell in the body is the sperm cell.

- Each cell in the body has its own energy plant, called the mitochondria.

- If all the capillaries were lined up end to end, they would encircle the earth at the equator 2 ½ times.

- For every pound of fat the body has to supply 200 miles of blood capillaries.

- It is through the circulation of the blood that each cell receives nutrients to perform its job, and to remove waste products.

Now that you know more about the body, can you see why you need a lot of nutrition for fuel, maintenance, and repair? You are the mayor of an amazing biological city, and each cell looks to you to provide it with life-giving nutrients.

If your cells could vote, would you be re-elected?

> The good Lord gave you a body that can stand most anything. It's your mind you have to convince.
>
> **Vincent Lombardi**

Dr. Simeons' Original Work

Here is an abridged version of Dr. Simeons' diet for those who prefer to follow the original 500 calorie diet. His diet is based on a theory of "calorie restriction". My version of the diet is based on a theory of "balanced blood sugar". Both versions work, based on my experience with hundreds of patients. Choose the version that makes most sense to you and fits your lifestyle.

> The older you get, the tougher it is to lose weight, because by then your body and your fat are really good friends.
>
> **Author Unknown**

Pounds and Inches
(Abridged)

by

A.T.W. Simeons, M.D.

The Nature of Obesity

Obesity a Disorder

As a basis for our discuss we postulate that obesity in all its many forms is due to an abnormal functioning of some part of the body; and that every ounce of abnormally accumulated fat is always the result of the same disorder of certain regulatory mechanisms. Persons suffering from this particular disorder will get fat regardless of whether they eat excessively, normally or less than normal. A person who is free of the disorder will never get fat, even if he frequently overeats.

Those in whom the disorder is severe will accumulate fat very rapidly, those in whom it is moderate will gradually increase in weight and those in whom it is mild may be able to keep their excess-weight stationary for long periods, in all these cases a loss of weight brought about by dieting, treatments with thyroid, appetite-reducing drugs, laxatives, violent exercise, massage, baths is only temporary and will be rapidly regained as soon as the reducing regimen is relaxed. The reason is simply that none of these measures corrects the basic disorder.

While there are great variations in the severity of obesity, we shall consider all the different forms in both sexes and at all ages as always being due to the same disorder. Variations in form would then be partly a matter of degree, partly an inherited bodily constitution and partly the result of a secondary involvement of endocrine glands such as the pituitary, the thyroid, the adrenals or the sex glands. On the other hand, we postulate that no deficiency of any of these glands can ever directly produce the common disorder known as obesity.

If this reasoning is correct, it follows that a treatment aimed at curing the disorder must be equally effective in both sexes, at all ages and in all forms of obesity. Unless this is so, we are entitled to harbor grave doubts as to whether a given treatment corrects the underlying disorder. Moreover, any claim that the disorder has been corrected must be substantiated by the ability of the patient to eat normally of any food he pleases without regaining abnormal fat after treatment. Only if these conditions are fulfilled can we legitimately speak of curing obesity rather than of reducing weight.

Our problem thus presents itself as an enquiry into the localization and the nature of the disorder which leads to obesity. The history of this enquiry is a long series of high hopes and bitter disappointments.

The History of Obesity

There was a time, not so long ago, when obesity was considered a sign of health and prosperity in man and of beauty, amorousness and fecundity in women. This attitude probably dates back to Neolithic times, about 8000 years ago, when for the first time in the history of culture man began to own property, domestic animals, arable land, houses, pottery and metal tools. Before that, with the possible exception of some races such as the Hottentots, obesity was almost non-existent, as it still is in all wild animals and most primitive races.

Today obesity is extremely common among all civilized races, because a disposition to the disorder can be inherited. Wherever abnormal fat was regarded as an asset, sexual selection tended to propagate the trait. It is only in very recent times that manifest obesity has lost some of its allure, though the cult of the outsize bust—always a sign of latent obesity—shows that the trend still lingers on.

The Significance of Regular Meats

In the early Neolithic times another change took place which may well account for the fact that today nearly all inherited dispositions sooner or later develop into manifest obesity. This change was the institution of regular meals. In pre-Neolithic times man ate only when he was hungry and only as much as he required to still the pangs of hunger. Moreover, much of his food was raw and all of it was unrefined. He roasted his meat, he did not boil it, as he had no pots, and what little he may have grubbed from the earth and picked from the trees he ate as he went along.

The whole structure of man's omnivorous digestive tract is, like that of an ape, rat or pig, adjusted to the continual nibbles of tidbits. It is not suited to occasional gorging as is, for instance, the intestine of the carnivorous cat family. Thus the institution of regular meals, particularly of food rendered rapidly assimilated, placed a great burden on modern man's ability to cope with large quantities of food suddenly pouring into his system from the intestinal tract.

The institution of regular meals meant that man had to eat more than his body required at the moment of eating so as to tide him over until the next meal. Food rendered easily digestible suddenly flooded his body with nourishment of which he was in no need at the moment. Somehow, somewhere this surplus had to be stored.

Three Kinds of Fat

In the human body we can distinguish three kinds of fat. The first is the structural fat which fills the gaps between various organs, a sort of packing material. Structural fat also performs such

115

important functions as bedding the kidneys in soft elastic tissue, protecting the coronary arteries and keeping the skin smooth and taut, it also provides the springy cushion of hard fat under the bones of the feet, without which we would be unable to walk.

The second type of fat is a normal reserve of fuel upon which the body can freely draw when the nutritional income from the intestinal tract is insufficient to meet the demand. Such normal reserves are localized all over the body. Fat is a substance which packs the highest caloric value into the smallest space so that normal reserves of fuel for muscular activity and the maintenance of body temperature can be most economically stored in this form. Both these types of fat, structural and reserve, are normal, and even if the body stocks them to capacity this can never be called obesity.

Subcutaneous

But there is a third type of fat which is entirely abnormal. It is the accumulation of such fat, and of such fat only, from which the overweight patient suffers. This abnormal fat is also a potential reserve of fuel, but unlike the normal reserves it is not available to the body in a nutritional emergency. It is, so to speak, locked away in a fixed deposit and is not kept in a current account, as are the normal reserves.

Visceral (in abdomen, around major organs.)

When an obese patient tries to reduce by starving himself, he will first lose his normal fat reserves. When these are exhausted he begins to burn up structural fat, and only as a last resort will the body yield its abnormal reserves, though by that time the patient usually feels so weak and hungry that the diet is abandoned. It is just for this reason that obese patients complain that when they diet they lose the wrong fat. They feel famished and tired and their face becomes drawn and haggard, but their belly, hips, thighs and upper arms show little improvement. The fat they have come to detest stays on and the fat they need to cover their bones gets less and less. Their skin wrinkles and they look old and miserable. And that is one of the most frustrating and depressing experiences a human being can have.

Injustice to the Obese

When, then, obese patients are accused of cheating, gluttony, lack of will power, greed and sexual complexes, the strong become indignant and decide that modern medicine is a fraud and its representatives fools, while the weak just give up the struggle in despair. In either case the result is the same: a further gain in weight, resignation to an abominable fate and the resolution at least to live tolerably the short span allotted to them—a fig for doctors and insurance companies.

Obese patients only feel physically well as long as they are stationary or gaining weight. They may feel guilty, owing to the lethargy and indolence always associated with obesity. They may feel ashamed of what they have been led to believe is a lack of control. They may feel horrified by the appearance of their nude body and the tightness of their clothes. But they have a primitive feeling of animal content which turns to misery and suffering as soon as they make a resolute attempt to reduce. For this there are sound reasons.

The groundwork of all happiness is health.

Leigh Hunt

In the first place, more caloric energy is required to keep a large body at a certain temperature than to heat a small body. Secondly, the muscular effort of moving a heavy body is greater than in the case of a light body. The muscular effort consumes Calories which must be provided by food. Thus, all other factors being equal, a fat person requires more food than a lean one. One might therefore reason that if a fat person eats only the additional food his body requires he should be able to keep his weight stationary. Yet every physician who has studied obese patients under rigorously controlled conditions knows that this is not true. Many obese patients actually gain weight on a diet which is calorically deficient for their basic needs. There must thus be some other mechanism at work.

Glandular Theories

At one time it was thought that this mechanism might be concerned with the sex glands. Such a connection was suggested by the fact that many juvenile obese patients show an under-development of the sex organs. The middle-aged spread in men and the tendency of many women to put on weight in the menopause seems to indicate a casual connection between diminishing sex function and overweight. Yet when highly active sex hormones become available, it was found that their administration had no affect whatsoever on obesity. The sex glands could therefore not be the seat of the disorder.

The Thyroid Gland

When it was discovered that the thyroid gland controls the rate at which body-fuel is consumed, it was thought that by administering thyroid gland to obese patients their abnormal fat deposits could be burned up more rapidly. This too proved to be entirely disappointing, because as we now know, these abnormal deposits take no part in the body's energy-turnover—they are inaccessibly locked away. Thyroid medication merely forces the body to consume its normal fat reserves, which are already depleted in obese patients, and then to break down structurally essential fat without touching the abnormal deposits. In this way a patient may be brought to the brink of starvation in spite of having a hundred pounds of fat to spare. Thus any weight-loss brought about by thyroid medication is always at the expense of fat of which the body is in dire need.

While the majority of obese patients have a perfectly normal thyroid gland and some even have an overactive thyroid, one also occasionally sees a case with a real thyroid deficiency. In such cases, treatment with thyroid brings about a small loss of weight, but this is not due to the loss of any abnormal fat. It is entirely the result of the elimination of a mucoid substance, called myxedema, which the body accumulates when there is a marked primary thyroid deficiency. Moreover, patients suffering only from a severe lack of thyroid hormone never become obese in the true sense. Possibly also the observation that normal persons – though not the obese – lose weight rapidly when their thyroid becomes overactive may have contributed to the false notion that thyroid deficiency and obesity are connected. Much misunderstanding about the supposed role of the thyroid gland in obesity is still met with, and it is now really high time that thyroid preparations be once and for all struck off the list of remedies for obesity. This is particularly so because giving thyroid gland to an obese patient whose thyroid is either normal or overactive, besides being useless, is decidedly dangerous.

The Pituitary Gland

The next gland to be falsely incriminated was the anterior lobe of the pituitary or hypothesis. This most important gland lies well protected in a bony capsule at the base of the skull. It has a vast number of functions in the body, among which is the regulation of all the other important endocrine glands. The fact that various signs of anterior pituitary deficiency are often associated with the obesity raised the hope that the seat of the disorder might be in this gland. But although a large number of pituitary hormones have been isolated and many extracts of the gland prepared, not a single one or any combination of such factors proved to be of any value in the treatment of obesity. Quite recently, however, a fat-mobilizing factor has been found in pituitary glands but it is still too early to say whether this factor is destined to play a role in the treatment of obesity.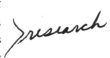

research

The Adrenals

Recently, a long series of brilliant discoveries concerning the working of the adrenal or suprarenal glands, small bodies which sit atop the kidneys, have created tremendous interest. This interest also turned to the problem of obesity when it was discovered that a condition which in some respects resembles a severe case of obesity—the so called Cushing's Syndrome—was caused by a glandular new-growth of the adrenals or by their excessive stimulation with ACTH, which is the pituitary hormone governing the activity of the outer rind or cortex of the adrenals.

When we learned that an abnormal stimulation of the adrenal cortex could produce signs that resemble true obesity, this knowledge furnished no practical means of treating obesity by decreasing the activity of the adrenal cortex. There is no evidence to suggest that in obesity there is any excess of adrenocortical activity; in fact, all the evidence points to the contrary. There seems to be rather a lack of adrenocortical functions and a decrease in the secretion of ACTH from the anterior pituitary lobe.

119

So here again our search for the mechanism which produces obesity led us into a blind alley. Recently, many students of obesity have reverted to the nihilistic attitude that obesity is caused simply by overeating and that it can only be cured by under eating.

The Diencephalon or Hypothalamus

For those of us who refused to be discouraged there remained one slight hope. Buried deep down in the massive human brain there is a part which we have in common with all vertebrate animals: the so-called diencephalon. It is a very primitive part of the brain and has in man been almost smothered by the huge masses of nervous tissue with which we think, reason and voluntarily move our body. The diencephalon is the part from which the central nervous system controls all the automatic animal functions of the body, such as breathing, the heartbeat, digestion, sleep, sex, the urinary system, the autonomous or vegetative nervous system and via the pituitary the whole interplay of the endocrine glands.

It was therefore not unreasonable to suppose that the complex operation of storing and issuing fuel to the body might also be controlled by the diencephalon. It has long been known that the content of sugar—another form of fuel—in the blood depends on a certain nervous center in the diencephalon. When this center is destroyed in laboratory animals they develop a condition rather similar to human stable diabetes. It has also long been known that the destruction of another diencephalic center produces a voracious appetite and a rapid gain in weight in animals which never get fat spontaneously.

The Fat-bank

Assuming that in a man such a center controlling the movement of fat does exist, its function would have to be much like that of a bank. When the body assimilates from the intestinal tract more fuel than it needs at the moment, this surplus is deposited in what may be compared with a current account. Out of this account it can it can always be withdrawn as required. All normal fat reserves are in such a current account, and it is probable that a diencephalic center manages the deposits and withdrawals.

When now, for reasons which will be discussed later, the deposits grow rapidly while small withdrawals become more frequent, a point may be reached which goes beyond the diencephalon's banking capacity. Just as a banker might suggest to a wealthy client that instead of accumulating a large and unmanageable current account he should invest his surplus capital, the body appears to establish a fixed deposit into which all surplus funds go but from which they can no longer be withdrawn by the procedure used in a current account. In this way the diencephalic "fat-bank" frees itself from all work which goes beyond its normal banking capacity. The onset of obesity dates from the moment the diencephalon adopts this laborsaving ruse. Once a fixed deposit has been established the normal fat reserves are held at a minimum, while every available surplus is locked away in the fixed deposit and is therefore taken out of normal circulation.

Pregnancy and Obesity

Once this trail was opened further observations seemed to fall into line. It is, for instance, well known that during pregnancy an obese woman can very easily lose weight. She can drastically reduce her diet without feeling hunger or discomfort and lose weight without harming the child in her womb. It is also surprising to what extent a woman can suffer from pregnancy vomiting without coming to any real harm.

Pregnancy is an obese woman's one great chance to reduce her excess weight. That she so rarely makes use of this opportunity is due to the erroneous notion, usually fostered by her elder relations, that she now has "two mouths to feed" and must "keep up her strength for the coming event." All modern obstetricians knows that this is nonsense and that the more superfluous fat is lost the less difficult will be the confinement, though some still hesitate to prescribe a diet sufficiently low in Calories to bring about a drastic reduction.

A woman may gain weight during pregnancy, but she never becomes obese in the strict sense of the word. Under the influence of the HCG which circulates in enormous quantities in her body during pregnancy, her diencephalic banking capacity seems to

Inside some of us is a thin person struggling to get out, but they can usually be sedated with a few pieces of chocolate cake.

Author Unknown

be unlimited, and abnormal fixed deposits are never formed. At confinement she is suddenly deprived of HCG, and her diencephalic fat-center reverts to its normal capacity. It is only then that the abnormally accumulated fat is locked away in a fixed deposit. From that moment on she is suffering from obesity and is subject to all its consequences.

Pregnancy seems to be the only normal human condition in which the diencephalic fat banking capacity is unlimited. It is only during pregnancy that fixed fat deposits can be transferred back into the normal current account and freely drawn upon to make up for any nutritional deficit. During pregnancy every ounce of reserve fat is placed at the disposal of the growing fetus. Were this not so, an obese woman, whose normal reserves are already depleted, would have the greatest difficulties in bringing her pregnancy to full term. There is considerable evidence to suggest that it is the HCG produced in large quantities in the placenta which brings about this diencephalic change.

Though we may be able to increase the diencephalic fat banking capacity by injecting HCG, this does not in itself affect the weight, just as transferring monetary funds from a fixed deposit into a current account does not make a man any poorer; to become poorer it is also necessary that he freely spend the money which thus becomes available. In pregnancy the needs of the growing embryo take care of this to some extent, but in the treatment of obesity there is no embryo, and so a very severe dietary restriction must take its place for the duration of treatment.

Only when the fat, which is in transit under the effect of HCG, is actually consumed can more fat be withdrawn from the fixed deposits. In pregnancy it would be most undesirable if the fetus were offered ample food only when there is a high influx from the intestinal tract. Ideal nutritional conditions for the fetus can only be achieved when the mother's blood is continually saturated with food, regardless of whether she eats or not, as otherwise a period of starvation might hamper the steady growth of the embryo. It seems that HCG brings about this continual saturation of the blood, which is the reason why obese patients under treatment with HCG never feel hungry in spite of their drastically reduced food intake.

HCG no Sex Hormone

It cannot be sufficiently emphasized that HCG is not sex- hormone, that its action is identical in men, women, children and in those cases in which the sex-glands no longer function owing to old age or their surgical removal. The only sexual change it can bring about after puberty is an improvement of a pre-existing deficiency. But never stimulation beyond the normal. In an indirect way, via the anterior pituitary, HCG regulates menstruation and facilitates conception, but it never virilizes a woman or feminizes a man. It neither makes men grow breasts nor does it interfere with their virility, though where this was deficient it may improve it. It never makes women grow a beard or develop a gruff voice. I have stressed this point only for the sake of my lay readers, because it is our daily experience that when patients hear the word "hormone" they immediately jump to the conclusion that this must have something to do with the sex-sphere. They are not accustomed as we are, to think of thyroid, insulin, cortisone, adrenalin etc, as hormones.

Gain before Loss

Patients whose general condition is low, owing to excessive previous dieting, must eat to capacity for about one week before starting treatment, regardless of how much weight they may gain in the process. One cannot keep a patient comfortably on 500 Calories unless his normal fat reserves are reasonably well stocked. It is for this reason also that every case, even those that are actually gaining must eat to capacity of the most fattening food they can get down until they have had their third injection. It is a fundamental mistake to put a patient on 500 Calories as soon as the injections are started, as it seems to take about three injections before abnormally deposited fat begins to circulate and thus become available.

We distinguish between the first three injections, which we call 'non-effective' as far as the loss of weight is concerned, and the subsequent injections given while the patient is dieting, which

123

we call "effective". The average loss of weight is calculated on the number of effective injections and from the weight reached on the day of the third injections which may be well above what it was two days earlier when the first injection was given.

Most patients who have been struggling with diets for years and know how rapidly they gain if they let themselves go are very hard to convince of the absolute necessity of gorging for at least two days, and yet this must be insisted upon categorically if the further course of treatment is to run smoothly. Those patients who have to be put on forced feeding for a week before starting the injections usually gain weight rapidly—four to six pounds in 24 hours is not unusual—but after a day or two this rapid gain generally levels off. In any case the whole gain is usually lost in the first 48 hours of dieting. It is necessary to proceed in this manner because the gain re-stocks the depleted normal reserves, whereas the subsequent loss is from the abnormal deposits only.

Patients in a satisfactory general condition and those who have not just previously restricted their diet start forced feeding on the day of the first injection. Some patents say that they can no longer overeat because their stomach has shrunk after years of restrictions. While we know that no stomach ever shrinks, we compromise by insisting that they eat frequently of highly concentrated foods such as milk chocolate, pastries with whipped cream sugar, fried meats particularly pork, eggs and bacon, mayonnaise, bread with thick butter and jam, etc. The time and trouble spent on pressing this point upon incredulous or reluctant patients is always amply rewarded afterwards by the complete absence of those difficulties which patients who have disregarded these instructions are liable to experience.

During the two days of forced feeding—from the first to the third injection—many patients are surprised that, contrary to their previous experience, they do not gain weight, and some even lose. The explanation is that in these cases there is a compensatory flow of urine, which drains excessive water from the body. To some extent this seems to be a direct action of HCG, but it may also be

500 Cal (handwritten)

due to a higher protein intake, as we know that a protein-deficient diet makes the body retain water.

Starting Treatment

In menstruating women the best time to start treatment is immediately after a period. Treatment may also be started later, but it is advisable to have at least ten days in hand before the onset of the next period.

The Diet

The 500 Calorie diet is explained on the day of the second injection to those patients who will be preparing their own food, and it is most important that the person who will actually cook is present – the wife, the mother or the cook, as the case may be. Here in Italy patients are given the following diet sheet.

Brain cells come and brain cells go, but fat cells live forever.

Author Unknown

BREAKFAST:

Tea or coffee in any quantity without sugar. Only one tablespoonful of milk allowed in 24 hours. Saccharin or other sweeteners may be used.

Fast or see next Pg (handwritten)

LUNCH:

3.5 oz (handwritten)

1. 100 grams of veal, beef, chicken breast, fresh white fish, lobster, crab, or shrimp. All visible fat must be carefully removed before cooking, and the meat must be weighed raw. It must be boiled or grilled without additional fat. Salmon, eel, tuna, herring, dried or pickled fish are not allowed. The chicken must be removed from the bird.

2. One type of vegetable only to be chosen from the following: spinach, chard, chicory, beet-greens, green salad, tomatoes, celery, fennel, onions, red radishes, cucumbers, asparagus, cabbage.

3. One bread stick (grissino) or one Melba toast.

4. An apple or an orange or a handful of strawberries or one-half grapefruit.

DINNER: The same four choices as lunch.

The juice of one lemon daily is allowed for all purposes. Salt, pepper, vinegar, mustard powder, garlic, sweet basil, parsley, thyme, marjoram, etc., may be used for seasoning, but no oil, butter or dressing.

Tea, coffee, plain water, mineral water are the only drinks allowed, but they may be taken in any quantity and at all times.

In fact the patient should drink about 2 liters of these fluids per day. Many patients are afraid to drink so much because they fear that this may make them retain more water. This is a wrong notion as the body is more inclined to store water when the intake falls below its normal requirements.

The fruit or the bread stick may be eaten between meals instead of with lunch or dinner, but not more than four items listed for lunch and dinner may be eaten at one meal.

No medicines or cosmetics other than lipstick, eyebrow pencil and powder may be used without special permission.

Every item in the list is gone over carefully, continually stressing the point that no variations other than those listed may be introduced. All things not listed are forbidden, and the patient is assured that nothing permissible has been left out. The 100 grams of meat must be scrupulously weighed raw after all visible fat has been removed. To do this accurately the patient must have a letter-scale, as kitchen scales are not sufficiently accurate and the butcher should certainly not be relied upon. Those not uncommon patients who feel that even so little food is too much for them, can omit anything they wish.

There is no objection to breaking up the two meals. For instance having a bread stick and an apple for breakfast or an orange before going to bed, provided they are deducted from the regular meals. The whole daily ration of two bread stick or two fruits may not be eaten at the same time, nor can any item saved from the previous day be added to the following day. In the beginning patients are advised to check every meal again on their diet sheet before starting to eat and not to rely on their memory. It is also worth pointing out that any attempt to observe this diet without HCG will lead to trouble in two or three days. We have had cases in which patients have proudly flaunted their dieting powers in front of their friends without mentioning the fact that they are also receiving treatment with HCG. They let their friends try the same diet, and when this proves to be a failure—as it necessarily must—the patient starts raking in unmerited kudos for superhuman willpower.

It should also be mentioned that two small apples weighing as much as one large one nevertheless have a higher caloric value and are therefore not allowed, though there is no restriction on the size of one apple. Some people do not realize that a tangerine is not an orange and that chicken breast does not mean the breast of any other fowl, nor does it mean a wing or drumstick.

The most tiresome patients are those who start counting Calories and then come up with all manner of ingenious variations, which they compile from their little books. When one has spent years of weary research trying to make a diet as attractive as possible without jeopardizing the loss of weight, culinary geniuses who are out to improve their unhappy lot are hard to take.

Making up the Calories

The diet used in conjunction with HCG must not exceed 500 Calories per day, and the way these Calories are made up is of utmost importance. For instance, if a patient drops the apple and eats an extra bread stick instead, he will not be getting more Calories but he will not lose weight. There are a number of foods, particularly fruits and vegetables, which have the same or even lower caloric values than those listed as permissible, and yet we find that they interfere with the regular loss of weight under HCG, presumably owing to the nature of their consumption. Pimiento peppers, okra, artichokes and pears are examples of this.

While this diet works satisfactory in Italy, certain modifications have to be made in other countries. For instance, American beef has almost double the caloric value of South Italian beef, which is not marbled with fat. This marbling is impossible to remove. In America, therefore, low-grade veal should be used for one meal and fish (excluding all those species such as herring, mackerel, tuna, salmon, eel, etc., which have high fat content, and all dried, smoked or pickled fish), chicken breast, lobster, crawfish, prawns, shrimps, crab meat or kidneys for the other meal. Where the Italian bread sticks, the so-called grissini, are not available, one Melba toast may be used instead, though they are psychologically less satisfying. A Melba toast has about the same weight as the very porous Grissini, which is much more to look at and to chew.

In many countries, specially prepared unsweetened and low Calorie foods are freely available, and some of these can be tentatively used. When local conditions or the feeding habits of the population make changes necessary it must be borne in mind that the total daily intake must not exceed 500 Calories if the best possible results are to be obtained, that the daily ration should contain 200 grams of fat-free protein and a very small amount of starch.

Just as the daily does of HCG is the same in all cases, so the same diet proves to be satisfactory for a small elderly lady of leisure or a hard working muscular giant. Under the effect of HCG the obese body is always able to obtain all the Calories it needs from the abnormal fat deposits, regardless of whether it uses up 1500 or 4000 per day. It must be made very clear to the patient that he is living to a far greater extent on the fat which he is losing than on what he eats.

Many patients ask why eggs are not allowed. The contents of two good-sized eggs are roughly equivalent to 100 grams of meat, but unfortunately the yolk contains a large amount of fat, which is undesirable. Very occasionally we allow egg—boiled, poached or raw—to patients who develop an aversion to meat, but in this case they must add the white of three eggs to the one they eat whole. In countries where cottage cheese made from skimmed milk is available 100 grams may occasionally be used instead of the meat, but no other cheeses are allowed.

Vegetarians

Strict vegetarians such as orthodox Hindus present a special problem, because milk and curds are the only animal protein they will eat. To supply them with sufficient protein of animal origin they must drink 500 cc. of skimmed milk per day, though part of this ration can be taken as curds. As far as fruit, vegetables and starch are concerned, their diet is the same as that of non-vegetarians; they cannot be allowed their usual intake of vegetable proteins from leguminous plants such as beans or from wheat or nuts, not can they have their customary rice. In spite of these severe restrictions, their average loss is about half that of non-vegetarians, presumably owing to the sugar content of the milk.

Faulty Dieting

Few patients will take one's word for it that the slightest deviation from the diet has under HCG disastrous results as far as the weight is concerned. This extreme sensitivity has the advantage that the smallest error is immediately detectable at the daily weighing but most patients have to have the experience before they will believe it.

Blessed are those who hunger and thirst, for they are sticking to their diets.

Anon

Persons in high official positions such as embassy personnel, politicians, senior executives, etc., who are obliged to attend social functions to which they cannot bring their meager meal must be told beforehand that an official dinner will cost them the loss of about three days treatment, however careful they are and in spite of a friendly and would-be cooperative host. We generally advise them to avoid all-round embarrassment, the almost inevitable turn of conversation to their weight problem and the outpouring of lay counsel from their table partners, by not letting it be known that they are under treatment. They should take dainty servings of everything, hide what they can under the cutlery and book the gain which may take three days to get rid of as one of the sacrifices which their profession entails. Allowing three days for their correction, such incidents do not jeopardize the treatment provided they do not occur too frequently, in which case treatment should be postponed to a socially more peaceful season.

Vitamins and Anemia

Sooner or later most patients express a fear that they may be running out of vitamins or that the restricted diet may make them anemic. On this score the physician can confidently relieve their apprehension by explaining that every time they lose a pound of fatty tissue, which they do almost daily, only the actual fat is burned up; all the vitamins, the proteins, the blood and the minerals which this tissue contains in abundance are fed back into the body. Actually, a low blood count not due to any serious disorder of the blood-forming tissues improves during treatment, and we have never encountered a significant protein deficiency or signs of lack of vitamins in patients who are dieting regularly.

The First Days of Treatment

On the day of the third injection it is almost routine to hear two remarks. One is: "You know, Doctor, I'm sure it's only psychological, but I already feel quite different". So common is this remark, even from very skeptical patients, that we hesitate to accept the psychological interpretation. The other typical remark is: "Now that I have been allowed to eat anything I want, I can't get it down. Since yesterday I feel like a stuffed pig. Food just doesn't seem to interest me anymore, and I am longing to get on with your diet". Many patients notice that they are passing more urine and that the swelling on their ankles is less even before they start dieting.

On the day of the fourth injection most patients declare that they are feeling fine. They have usually lost two pounds or more, some say they feel a bit empty but hasten to explain that this does not amount to hunger. Some complain of a mild headache of which they have been forewarned and for which they have been given permission to take aspirin.

During the second and third day or dieting—that is, the fifth and sixth injection—these minor complaints improve while the weight continues to drop at about double the usual overall average of almost one pound per day, so that a moderately severe case may by the fourth day of dieting have lost as much as 8-10 lbs.

It is usually at this point that a difference appears between those patients who have literally eaten to capacity during the first two days of treatment and those who have not. The former feel remarkably well; they have no hunger, nor do they feel tempted when others eat normally at the table. They feel lighter, more clear-headed and notice a desire to move quite contrary to their previous lethargy. Those who have disregarded the advice to eat to capacity continue to have minor discomforts and do not have the same euphoric sense of self-being until about a week later. It seems that their normal fat reserves require that much more time before they are fully stocked.

Fluctuations in Weight Loss

After the fourth or fifth day of dieting the daily loss of weight begins to decrease to one pound or somewhat less per day, and there is a smaller urinary output. Men often continue to lose regularly at that rate, but women are more irregular in spite of faultless dieting. There may be no drop at all for two or three days and then a sudden loss which reestablishes the normal average. These fluctuations are entirely due to variations in the retention and elimination of water, which are more marked in women than in men.

The weight registered by the scale is determined by two processes, not necessarily synchronized. Under the influence of HCG, fat is being extracted from the cells in which it is stored in the fatty tissue. When these cells are empty and therefore serve no purpose the body breaks down the cellular structure and absorbs it, but breaking up of useless cells, connective tissue, blood vessels, etc., may lag behind the process of fat-extraction. When this happens, the body appears to replace some of the extracted fat with water which is retained for this purpose. As water is heavier than fat the scales may show no loss of weight, although sufficient fat has actually been consumed to make up for the deficit in the 500 Calorie diet. When such tissue is finally broken down, the water is liberated and there is a sudden flood of urine and a marked loss of weight. This simple interpretation of what is really an extremely complex mechanism is the one we give those patients who want to know why it is that on certain days they do not lose, though they have committed no dietary error.

Patients who have previously regularly used diuretics as a method of reducing may lose fat during the first two or three weeks of treatment which shows in their measurements, but the scale may show little or no loss because they are replacing the normal water content of their body, which has been dehydrated. Diuretics should never be used for reducing.

Interruptions of Weight Loss

We distinguish four types of interruption in the regular daily loss. The first is the one that has already been mentioned, in which the weight stays stationary for a day or two, and this occurs, particularly towards the end of a course, in almost every case.

The Plateau

The second type of interruption we call a "plateau." A plateau lasts 4-6 days and frequently occurs during the second half of a full course, particularly in patients that have been doing well and whose overall average of nearly a pound per effective injection has been maintained. Those who are losing more than the average all have a plateau sooner or later. A plateau always corrects itself, but many patients who have become accustomed to a regular daily loss get unnecessarily worried and begin to fret. No amount of explanation convinces them that a plateau does not mean that they are no longer responding normally to treatment.

In such cases we consider it permissible, for purely psychological reasons, to break up the plateau. This can be done in two ways. One is a so-called "apple day". An apple day begins at lunch and continues until just before lunch of the following day. The patients are given six large apples and are told to eat one whenever they feel the desire though six apples is the maximum allowed. During an apple-day no other food or liquids except plain water are allowed, and of water they may only drink just enough to quench an uncomfortable thirst if eating an apple still leaves them thirsty. Most patients feel no need for water and are quite happy with their six apples. Needless to say, an apple day may never be given on the day on which there is no injection. The apple day produces a gratifying loss of weight on the following day, chiefly due to the elimination of water. The water is not regained when the patients resume their normal 500 Calorie diet at lunch, and on the following days they continue to lose weight satisfactorily.

The other way to break up a plateau is by giving a non-mercurial diuretic for one day. This is simpler for the patient but we prefer the apple-day as we sometimes find that though the diuretic is very effective on the following day, it may take two to three days before the normal daily reduction is resumed, throwing the patient into a new fit of despair. It is useless to give either an apple-day or diuretic unless the weight has been stationary for at least four days without any dietary error having been committed.

Reaching a Former Level

The third type of interruption in the regular loss of weight may last much longer—ten days to two weeks. Fortunately, it is rare and only occurs in very advanced cases, and then hardly ever during the first course of treatment. It is seen only in those patients who during some period of their lives have maintained a certain fixed degree of obesity for ten years or more and have then at some time rapidly increased beyond the weight. When, in the course of treatment, the former level is reached, it may take two weeks of no loss, in spite of HCG and diet, before further reduction is normally resumed.

The road to success is dotted with many tempting parking places.

Anon

Menstrual Interruption

The fourth type of interruption is the one which often occurs a few days before and during the menstrual period and in some women at the time of ovulation. It must also be mentioned that when a woman becomes pregnant during treatment- and this is by no means uncommon – she at once ceases to lose weight. An unexplained arrest of reduction has on several occasions raised our suspicion before the first period was missed. If in such cases menstruation is delayed, we stop injecting and do a precipitation test five days later. No pregnancy test should be carried out earlier than five days after the last injection, as otherwise the HCG may give a false positive result.

Oral contraceptives may be used during treatment.

Cosmetics

When no dietary error is elicited we turn to cosmetics. Most women find it hard to believe that fats, oils, creams and ointments applied to the skin are absorbed and interfere with weight reduction by HCG just as if they had been eaten. This almost incredible sensitivity to even such very minor increases in nutritional intake is a peculiar feature of the HCG method. For instance, we find that persons who habitually handle organic fats, such as workers in beauty parlors, masseurs, butchers, etc. never show what we consider a satisfactory loss of weight unless they can avoid fat coming into contact with their skin.

The point is so important that I will illustrate it with two cases. A lady who was cooperating perfectly suddenly increased half a pound. Careful questioning brought nothing to light. She had certainly made no dietary error nor had she used any kind of face cream, and she was already in the menopause. As we felt that we could trust her implicitly, we left the question suspended. Yet just as she was about to leave the consulting worn she suddenly stopped, turned and snapped her fingers. "I've got it" she said. This is what had happened: She had brought herself a new set of make-up pots and bottles and, using her fingers, had transferred her large assortment of cosmetics to the new containers in anticipation of the day she would be able to use them again after her treatment.

The other case concerns a man who impressed us as being very conscientious. He was about 20 lbs. overweight but did not lose satisfactorily from the onset of treatment. Again and again we tried to find the reason but with no success, until one day he said: "I never told you this, but I have a glass eye. In fact, I have a whole set of them. I frequently change them, and every time I do that I put a special ointment in my eye socket. Do you think that could have anything to do with it?" As we thought just that, we asked him to stop using this ointment, and from that day on his weight-loss was regular.

We are particularly averse to those modern cosmetics that contain hormones, as any interference with endocrine regulations during treatment must be absolutely avoided. Many women whose skin has in the course of years become adjusted to the use of fat-containing cosmetics find that their skin gets dry as soon as they stop using them. In such cases we permit the use of plain mineral oil, which has no nutritional value. On the other hand, mineral oil should not be used in preparing food, first because of its undesirable laxative quality, and second because it absorbs some fat-soluble vitamins, which are then lost in the stool. We do permit the use of lipstick, powder and such lotions as are entirely free of fatty substances. We also allow brilliantine to be used on the hair, but it must not be rubbed into the scalp. Obviously suntan oil is prohibited.

Many women are horrified when told that for the duration of treatment they cannot use face creams or have facial massages. They fear that this and the loss of weight will ruin their complexion. They can be fully reassured. Under treatment normal fat is restored to the skin, which rapidly becomes fresh and turgid, making the expression more youthful. This is a characteristic of the HCG method, which is a constant source of wonder to patients who have experienced or seen in others the facial ravages produced by the usual methods of reducing. An obese woman of 70 obviously cannot expect to have her puffed face reduced to normal without a wrinkle, but it is remarkable how youthful her face remains in spite of her age.

The Voice

Incidentally, another interesting feature of the HCG method is that it does not ruin a singing voice. The typically obese prima donna usually finds that, when she tries to reduce, the timbre of her voice is liable to change, and understandably this terrifies her. Under HCG this does not happen; indeed, in many cases the voice improves and the breathing invariably does. We have had many cases of professional singers very carefully controlled by expert voice teachers, and the maestros have been so enthusiastic that they now frequently send us patients.

Other reasons for a Gain

Apart from diet and cosmetics there can be a few other reasons for a small rise in weight. Some patients unwittingly take chewing gum, throat pastilles, vitamin pills, cough syrups, etc., without realizing that the sugar or fats they contain may interfere with a regular loss of weight. Sex hormones or cortisone in its various modern forms must be avoided, though oral contraceptives are permitted. In fact the only self-medication we allow is aspirin for a headache, though headaches almost invariably disappear after a week of treatment, particularly if of the migraine type.

Occasionally we allow a sleeping table or a tranquilizer, but patients should be told that while under treatment they need and may get less sleep. For instance, here in Italy where it is customary to sleep during the siesta, which lasts from one to four in the afternoon, most patients find that though they lie down they are unable to sleep.

We encourage swimming and sun bathing during the treatment, but it should be remembered that a severe sunburn always produces a temporary rise in weight, evidently due to water retention. The same may be seen when a patient gets a common cold during treatment. Finally, the weight can temporarily increase—paradoxical though this may sound—after an exceptional physical exertion of long duration leading to a feeling of exhaustion. A game of tennis, a vigorous swim, a run, a ride on horseback or a round of golf do not have this effect; but a long trek, a day of skiing, rowing or cycling or dancing into the small hours usually results in a gain of weight on the following day, unless the patient is in perfect training. In patients coming from abroad, where they always use their cars, we often see this effect after a strenuous day of shopping on foot, sightseeing and visits to galleries and museums. Though the extra muscular effort involved does consume some additional Calories, this appears to be offset by the retention of water, which the tired circulation cannot at once eliminate.

Blood Sugar

Towards the end of a course or when a patient has nearly reached his normal weight it occasionally happens that the blood sugar drops below normal, and we have even seen this in patients who had an abnormally high blood sugar before treatment. Such an attack of hypoglycemia is almost identical with the one seen in diabetics who have taken too much insulin. The attack comes on suddenly, there is the same feeling of light-headedness, weakness in the knees, trembling and unmotivated sweating; but under HCG hypoglycemia does not produce any feeling of hunger. All these symptoms are almost instantly relieved by taking two heaped teaspoonfuls of sugar.

In the course of treatment the possibility of such an attack is explained to those patients who are in a phase in which a drop in blood sugar may occur. They are instructed to keep sugar or glucose sweets handy, particularly when driving a car. They are also held to watch the effect of taking sugar very carefully and report the following day. This is important, because anxious patients to whom such an attack has been explained are apt to take sugar unnecessarily, in which case it inevitably produces a gain in weight and does not dramatically relieve the symptoms for which it was taken, proving that these were not due to hypoglycemia. Some patients mistake the effects of emotional stress for hypoglycemia. When the symptoms are quickly relieved by sugar this is proof that they were indeed due to an abnormal lowering of the blood sugar, and in that case there is no increase in the weight on the following day. We always suggest that sugar be taken if the patient is in doubt.

Once such an attack has been relieved with sugar we have never seen it recur on the immediately subsequent days, and only very rarely does a patient have two such attacks separated by several days during a course of treatment.

> In general, mankind, since the improvement of cookery, eats twice as much as nature requires.
>
> **Benjamin Franklin**

The Ratio of Pounds to Inches

An interesting feature of the HCG method is that, regardless of how fat a patient is, the greatest circumference—abdomen or hips as the case may be—is reduced at a constant rate which is extraordinarily close to 1 cm. per kilogram of weight lost. At the beginning of treatment the change in measurements is somewhat greater than this, but at the end of a course it is almost invariably found that the girth is as many centimeters less as the number or kilograms by which the weight has been reduced. I have never seen this clear-cut relationship in patients that try to reduce by dieting only.

Fibroids

While uterine fibroids seem to be in no way affected by HCG in the doses we use, we have found that very large, externally palpable uterine myomas are apt to give trouble. We are convinced that this is entirely due to the rather sudden disappearance of fat from the pelvic bed upon which they rest, and that it is the weight of the tumor pressing on the underlying tissues which accounts for the discomfort or pain which may arise during treatment. While we disregard even fair-sized or multiple myomas, we insist that very large ones be operated before treatment. We have had patients present themselves for reducing fat from their abdomen who showed no signs of obesity, but had a large abdominal tumor.

Gallstones

Small stones in the gall bladder may, in patients who have recently had typical colics, cause more frequent colics under treatment with HCG. This may be due to the almost complete absence of fat from the diet, which prevents the normal emptying of the gall bladder. Before undertaking treatment we explain to such patients that there is a risk of more frequent and possibly severe symptoms and that it may become necessary to operate. If they are prepared to take this risk and provided they agree to undergo an operation if we consider this imperative we proceed with treatment as after weight reduction with HCG the operative risk is considerably reduced in an obese patient. In such cases we always give a drug which stimulates the flow of bile, and in the majority of cases nothing untoward happens. On the other hand, we have looked for and not found any evidence to suggest that the HCG treatment leads to the formation of gallstones as pregnancy sometimes does.

The Heart

Disorders of the heart are not as a rule contraindications. In fact, the removal of abnormal fat—particularly from the heart muscle and from the surrounding of the coronary arteries— can only be beneficial in cases of myocardial weakness, and many such patients are referred to us by cardiologists. Within the first week of treatment all patients—not only heart cases—remark that they have lost much of their breathlessness.

Coronary Occlusion

In obese patients who have recently survived a coronary occlusion we adopt the following procedure in collaboration with the cardiologist. We wait until no further electrocardiographic changes have occurred for a period of three months. Routine treatment is then started under careful control and it is usual to find a further electrocardiographic improvement of a condition which was previously stationary.

In thousands of cases we have treated we have not once seen any sort of coronary incident occur during or shortly after treatment. The same applies to cerebral vascular accidents. Nor have we ever seen a case of thrombosis of any sort develop during treatment, even though a high blood pressure is rapidly lowered. In this respect, too, the HCG treatment resembles pregnancy.

Teeth and Vitamins

Patients whose teeth are in poor repair sometimes get more trouble under prolonged treatment, just as may occur in pregnancy. In such cases we do allow calcium and vitamin D, though not in an oily solution. The only other vitamin we permit is vitamin C, which we use in large doses combined with an antihistamine at the onset of a common cold. There is no objection to the use of an antibiotic if this is required, for instance by the dentist. In cases of bronchial asthma and hay fever we have occasionally resorted to cortisone during treatment and find that triamcinolone is the least likely to interfere with the loss of weight, but many asthmatics improve with HCG alone.

Alcohol

Obese heavy drinkers, even those bordering on alcoholism, often do surprisingly well under HCG and it is exceptional for them to take a drink while under treatment. When they do, they find that a relatively small quantity of alcohol produces intoxication. Such patients say that they do not feel the need to drink. This may in part be due to the euphoria which the treatment produces and in part to the complete absence of the need for a quick sustenance from which most obese patients suffer.

Though we have had a few cases that have continued abstinence long after treatment, others relapse as soon as they are back on a normal diet. We have a few "regular customers" who, having once been reduced to their normal weight, start to drink again though watching their weight. Then after some months they purposely overeat in order to gain sufficient weight for another course of HCG which temporarily gets them out of their drinking routine.

We do not particularly welcome such cases, but we see no reason for refusing their request.

Tuberculosis

It is interesting that obese patients suffering from inactive pulmonary tuberculosis can be safely treated. We have under very careful control treated patients as early as three months after they were pronounced inactive and have never seen a relapse occur during or shortly after treatment. In fact, we only have one case on our records in which active tuberculosis developed in a young man about one year after a treatment which had lasted three weeks. Earlier X-rays showed a calcified spot from a childhood infection which had not produced clinical symptoms. There was a family history of tuberculosis, and his illness started under adverse conditions which certainly had nothing to do with the treatment. Residual calcifications from an early infection are exceedingly common, and we never consider them a contraindication to treatment.

The Painful Heel

In obese patients who have been trying desperately to keep their weight down by severe dieting, a curious symptom sometimes occurs. They complain of an unbearable pain in their heels which they feel only while standing or walking. As soon as they take the weight off their heels the pain ceases. These cases are the bane of the rheumatologists and orthopedic surgeons who have treated them before they come to us. All the usual investigations are entirely negative, and there is not the slightest response to anti-rheumatic medication or physiotherapy. The pain may be so severe that the patients are obliged to give up their occupation, and they are not infrequently labeled as a case of hysteria. When their heels are carefully examined one finds that the sole is softer than normal and that the heel bone—the calcaneus—can be distinctly felt, which is not the case in a normal foot.

We interpret the condition as a lack of the hard fatty pad on which the calcaneus rests and which protects both the bone and the skin of the sole from pressure. This fat is like a springy cushion which carries the weight of the body. Standing on a heel in which this fat is missing or reduced must obviously be very painful. In their efforts to keep their weight down these patients have consumed this normal structural fat.

Those patients who have a normal or subnormal weight while showing the typically obese fat deposits are made to eat to capacity, often much against their will, for one week. They gain weight rapidly but there is no improvement in the painful heels. They are then started on the routine HCG treatment. Overweight patients are treated immediately. In both cases the pain completely disappears in 10-20 days of dieting, usually around the 15th day of treatment, and so far no case has had a relapse, though we have been able to follow up such patients for years.

We are particularly interested in these cases, as they furnish further proof of the contention that HCG + 500 Calories not only removes abnormal fat but actually permits normal fat to be replaced, in spite of the deficient food intake. It is certainly not so that the mere loss of weight reduces the pain, because it frequently disappears before the weight the patient had prior to the period of forced feeding is reached.

> As for food, half of my friends have dug their graves with their teeth.
>
> **Chauncey M. Depew**

Concluding a Course

When the three days of dieting after the last injection are over, the patients are told that they may now eat anything they please, except sugar and starch, provided they faithfully observe one simple rule. This rule is that they must have their own portable bathroom-scale always at hand, particularly while traveling. They must without fail weigh themselves every morning as they get out of bed, having first emptied their bladder. If they are in the habit of having breakfast in bed, they must weigh before breakfast.

It takes about 3 weeks before the weight reached at the end of the treatment becomes stable, i.e. does not show violent fluctuations after an occasional excess. During this period patients must realize that the so-called carbohydrates, that is sugar, rice, bread, potatoes, pastries, etc., are by far the most dangerous. A small quantity of alcohol, such as a glass of wine with meals, does no harm, but as soon as fats and starch are combined things are very liable to get out of hand. This has to be observed very carefully during the first

3 weeks after the treatment is ended otherwise disappointments are almost sure to occur.

Skipping a Meal

As long as their weight stays within two pounds of the weight reached on the day of the last injection, patients should take no notice of any increase but the moment the scale goes beyond two pounds, even if this is only a few ounces, they must on that same day entirely skip breakfast and lunch but take plenty to drink. In the evening they must eat a huge steak with only an apple or raw tomato. Of course this rule applies only to the morning weight. Ex-obese patients should never check their weight during the day, as there may be wide fluctuations and these are merely alarming and confusing.

It is of utmost importance that the meal is skipped on the same day as the scale registers an increase of more than two pounds and that missing the meals is not postponed until the following day. If a meal is skipped on the day in which a gain is registered in the morning this brings about an immediate drop of often over a pound. But if the skipping of the meal— and skipping means literally skipping not just having a light meal—is postponed the phenomenon does not occur, and several days of strict dieting may be necessary to correct the situation.

Most patients hardly ever need to skip a meal. If they have eaten a heavy lunch they feel no desire to eat their dinner, and in this case no increase takes place. If they keep their weight at the point reached at the end of the treatment, even a heavy dinner does not bring about an increase of two pounds on the next morning and does not therefore call for any special measures. Most patients are surprised how small their appetite has become and yet how much they can eat without gaining weight. They no longer suffer from an abnormal appetite and feel satisfied with much less food than before. In fact, they are usually disappointed that they cannot manage their first normal meal, which they have been planning for weeks.

Losing More Weight

An ex-patient should never gain more than two pounds without immediately correcting this, but it is equally undesirable that more than two lbs. be lost after treatment, because a greater loss is always achieved at the expense of normal fat. Any normal fat that is lost is invariably regained as soon as more food is taken, and it often happens that this rebound overshoots the upper two lbs. limit.

Trouble After Treatment

Two difficulties may be encountered in the immediate post treatment period. When a patient has consumed all his abnormal fat or when, after a full course, the injection has temporarily lost its efficacy owing to the body having gradually evolved a counter regulation, the patient at once begins to feel much more hungry and even weak. In spite of repeated warning, some over-enthusiastic patients do not report this. However, in about two days the fact that they are being undernourished becomes visible in their faces, and treatment is then stopped at once. In such cases—and only in such cases—we allow a very slight increase in the diet, such as an extra apple, 150 grams of meat or two or three extra bread sticks during the three days of dieting after the last injection.

When abnormal fat is no longer being put into circulation, either because it has been consumed or because immunity has set in, this is always felt by the patient as sudden, intolerable and constant hunger. In this sense the HCG method is completely self-limiting. With HCG it is impossible to reduce a patient, however enthusiastic, beyond his normal weight. As soon as no more abnormal fat is being issued the body starts consuming normal fat, and this is always regained as soon as ordinary feeding is resumed. The patient then finds that the 2–3 lbs. he has lost during the last days of treatment are immediately regained. A meal is skipped and maybe a pound is lost. The next day this pound is regained, in spite of a careful watch over the food intake. In a few days a tearful patient is back in the consulting room, convinced that her case is a failure.

All that is happening is that the essential fat lost at the end of the treatment, owing to the patient's reluctance to report a much greater hunger, is being replaced. The weight at which such a patient must stabilize thus lies 2-3 lbs. higher than the weight reached at the end of treatment. Once this higher basic level is established, further difficulties in controlling the weight at the new point of stabilization hardly arise.

Beware of Over-enthusiasm

The other trouble which is frequently encountered immediately after treatment is again due to over-enthusiasm. Some patients cannot believe that they can eat fairly normally without regaining weight. They disregard the advice to eat anything they please except sugar and starch and want to play safe. They try more or less to continue the 500 Calorie diet on which they felt so well during treatment and make only minor variations, such as replacing the meat with an egg, cheese or a glass of milk. To their horror they find that in spite of this bravura their weight goes up. So, following instructions, they skip one meager lunch and at night eat only a little salad and drink a pot of unsweetened tea, becoming increasingly hungry and weak. The next morning they find that they have increased yet another pound. They feel horrible, and even the dreaded swelling of their ankles is back. Normally we check our patients one week after they have been eating freely, but these cases return in a few days. Either their eyes are filled with tears or they angrily imply that when we told them to eat normally we were just fooling them.

Protein Deficiency

Here too, the explanation is quite simple. During treatment the patient has been only just above the verge of protein deficiency and has had the advantage of protein being fed back into his system from the breakdown of fatty tissue. Once the treatment is over there is no more HCG in the body and this process no longer takes place. Unless an adequate amount of protein is eaten as soon as the treatment is over, protein deficiency is bound to develop, and this inevitably causes the marked retention of water known as hunger edema.

The treatment is very simple. The patient is told to eat two eggs for breakfast and a huge steak for lunch and dinner followed by a large helping of cheese and to phone though the weight the next morning. When these instructions are followed a stunned voice is heard to report that two lbs. have vanished overnight, that the ankles are normal but that sleep was disturbed, owing to an extraordinary need to pass large quantities of water. The patient having learned this lesson usually has no further trouble.

Relapses

As a general rule one can say that 60%-70% of our cases experience little or no difficulty in holding their weight permanently. Relapses may be due to negligence in the basic rule of daily weighing. Many patients think that this is unnecessary and that they can judge any increase from the fit of their clothes. Some do not carry their scale with them on a journey as it is cumbersome and takes a big bite out of their luggage-allowance when flying. This is a disastrous mistake, because after a course of HCG as much as 10 lbs. can be regained without any noticeable change in the fit of the clothes. The reason for this is that after treatment newly acquired fat is at first evenly distributed and does not show the former preference for certain parts of the body.

If hunger is not the problem, then eating is not the solution.

Author Unknown

Real Questions From Patients and Clients

On bingeing, can I binge on good food? I hate to throw crap in my body. I eat very well now, almost like the diet except larger portions. Of course I indulge in sushi and ice cream, my favorite indulges, once in awhile. That's why I want to try this diet, because I eat so well and still can't lose weight.

Yes, fatty foods like cheese, avocado and ice cream are fine. The idea is to get some fat in circulation.

Won't the released fat go to my arteries and be dangerous for my heart?

No, the fat that is released will be used for fuel for your muscles. By the way, it is not fat in arteries that causes problems, but plaque build-up. Even this is controversial, according to studies. Some people who have great plaque build-up that shows up at autopsy do not die of heart attacks. Other people die of heart attacks with no plaque build-up. See "Good Calories, Bad Calories" by Gary Taubes for more information on the relationship between diet, obesity and heart disease.

The 6 oz of meat for lunch or dinner, is that 6 oz BEFORE or AFTER cooking?

You don't need to be too concerned on the FAT FIX DIET, because it is about blood sugar balance, but usually best to measure before.

The biggest seller is cookbooks and the second is diet books – how not to eat what you've just learned how to cook.

Andy Rooney

147

The egg white omelet listed for breakfast, which I will probably eat for lunch, how many eggs is the limit?

2-3 egg whites. 1/2 cup skim cottage cheese is also allowed, but only a couple times a week.

Vegetables—what is the portion for lunch and dinner?

No real limit. It is hard to overeat veggies if no oil or butter is used.

A friend of mine wants to try the diet but has a very high lipid count and very high cholesterol so she is concerned that the fat breaking down and entering the blood stream could be harmful to her heart. What do you think?

There is dietary fat in the bloodstream all the time. When you eat any fat, or any food at all, it breaks down into tiny "bits" in the intestine and is absorbed into the system and eventually makes it's way to the muscles for fuel and to cell membranes, which are formed out of "lipids" or fats. Fatty acids, which make up fats are absolutely vital for human health! It is really sugar that increases heart risk, not dietary fat. Sugar is converted into triglycerides in the liver, which raise cholesterol and triglyceride levels in the blood. Want to decrease your heart disease risk? Eat good fats like virgin olive oil and organic butter and eliminate white flour and sugars. 90% of the fat in red meat is the same type of fat that is in olive oil.

The fat tissue that is broken down by the homeopathic HCG will be used by the body for fuel, mainly by the muscles. Your body will not release more fat than it can use at the time, so this program is very heart healthy.

I am only 10 pounds overweight so I only want to do for 2 weeks is that OK?

It is better to do the program for at least 3 weeks. You won't lose more weight than you need to, but you will help the body to take on more of a fat burning mode. Two weeks is not really long enough for your body to make the full change. This was the conclusion of Dr. Simeons.

Can I have two different vegetables at once?

Most people seem to lose weight mixing their vegetables. If you run into a plateau you can cut back to one vegetable at a time and see if that makes a difference for you.

From your personal experience and feedback, do you recommend doing mild exercise while on the program? I was a bit apprehensive as I thought that might make me more hungry.

Yes, I do recommend mild exercise. You can still lose weight doing no exercise, but I think the body was designed to move around. Studies have shown there is less risk of heart problems if people move. Most of us live sedentary life-styles and it is not healthy. Try walking ½ hour per day, or doing Pilates or Yoga.

Quick question, do the homeopathic hcg drops have an expiration date? Just wondering as I'm starting back up and didn't finish my previous bottle so was planning to use those until they ran out.

Homeopathic remedies are very stable at room temperature. There is a small amount of alcohol in the Magic Drops, so you don't have to worry about expiration for a very long time. The glass bottle is dark to protect from light. You don't have to refrigerate the drops, but keep them out of extreme temperatures, and away from direct sunlight. If you prefer not to have any alcohol at all, put the drops into a small amount of boiling water for a minute. Remove from stove and let cool and the alcohol will dissipate. Then drink the water. Hold under your tongue just as you do the Drops.

I'm currently using a vaginal hormone cream that has really helped to keep my hormones in check during menopause and I've come to rely on it.

Just want to make sure that this will not interfere with the other hormones that I'm now taking.

There should not be a problem with continuing your hormonal creams.

I have one of those foot detox machines. Is that allowed during the diet?

Yes, it is okay to use the ionic foot machine. Be sure to drink plenty of water afterwards, to avoid dehydration.

On the paperwork it gives different lengths of time of doing the diet but some of the other diets see to go for 40 days. What is the correct way to do it?

I'm guessing it depends on how much you want to lose, right?

Yes, you may choose a 3, 4 or 6 week program. It is not a good idea to do one round beyond 6-7 weeks. Your body needs some dietary fat to help the gall bladder to function normally. The gall bladder contracts and releases bile when you eat fat. Do a strict Maintenance and then do another full round of the FAT FIX DIET to lose more weight.

How many days is the bottle for that we have?

The 2 oz. bottle should last you 4 weeks.

What is considered strenuous exercise? Like weight lifting, aerobics, or running? I usually lift heavy weights twice a week, take an aerobics class twice, and run twice a week, do yoga at least once, and try to walk about 2 miles in the evening. Perhaps I should just do my 2 mile walks and yoga or... ????

Walking, Pilates, Yoga, etc. is all you should do when taking the Magic Drops or any other kind of HCG. On the Maintenance phase you can go back to a heavier workout. I am a little confused on the amount of food- so I remember you saying you can have up to 6 oz protein but the standard amount is 3.5 oz, weighed raw- right? Then on the servings of vegetables you just have whatever calories worth you have left?

If you are following Dr. Simeons' protocol you can eat only 100 grams or 3 oz. of protein (weighed before cooking) twice a day. On the Fat Fix Diet plan you can eat 6 oz. of protein at a time. Dr. Simeons' program is based on calorie deprivation and mine is based on blood sugar balance. Best to measure before cooking, but if you are eating out, you will have to "guesstimate".

> I go up and down the scale so often that if they ever perform an autopsy on me they'll find me like a strip of bacon - a streak of lean and a streak of fat.
>
> **Texas Guinan**

How long should I wait before starting the diet again?

Dr. Simeons recommended waiting for as many weeks as you did his diet; 3 weeks of diet = 3 weeks wait, etc. With the homeopathic HCG you can wait just 3 weeks between each round. Be sure to do the Maintenance strictly to reset your metabolism and set your new lower weight.

However for later rounds, it does seem it is better to wait longer between. If you plan to do a third round, it may be a good idea to wait 5-6 weeks between. If you stay on the Maintenance fairly strictly you can maintain your loss and possibly even lose more. The biggest mistake people make is to let old habits creep in. Do a "steak day" is you gain two pounds and stay on top of the weight loss.

Often people find they lose more inches than pounds in later rounds and the weight loss slows down. One of the distributors who has maintained a 50 pound loss after her full FAT FIX DIET program suggests just hanging in and persisting if the body seems to resist dropping weight. Staying strong and disciplined is the key. There are different body types and not every body is meant to be skinny. But I don't believe that anyone is genetically programmed to be obese, either.

Some people find that their body is better than ever with the program and using the Magic Drops. Their body seems to find its true shape, even after age 60.

If I were to take the drops 4 times a day would it benefit me in any way? I'm sometimes only losing .2 or .4 of a pound and I still have quite a bit I want to lose. Some days it's a whole pound which I prefer of course ;)

Yes, some people can do well using the Magic Drops 4 times a day. You can also try this to break a plateau or help with hunger.

Or is there anything else I can do to speed it up or would help?

Do some walking or light exercise. You could walk 20-30 minutes twice a day and that might help.

The diet lets me eat applies, oranges, grapefruit, etc. But nowhere does it say I can drink apple juice, orange juice, grapefruit juice, etc. If I can eat an apple, what is the difference with drinking apple juice? Brands like "Simply Apple", etc., are 100% juice, with nothing added, and Bristol Farms sells 100% freshly squeezed orange juice. Can you tell me why it would be OK to eat the fruit, but not drink the juice? Or put the fresh apples or oranges in my juicer and make juice?

No juice of any kind is allowed on the FAT FIX DIET because juice is a processed food. Fruit sugar gets converted into triglycerides and cholesterol faster than glucose or table sugar. The reason fruit is allowed is because the fiber in the fruit slows down the release of fruit sugar. Unlimited fruit is not allowed, though, because that can increase your blood sugar levels and stop the action of the Homeopathic HCG.

I am a vegetarian. Can I do the FAT FIX DIET?

Yes, you can do a modified version. Please understand that you may not lose at the same rate as those who follow the original diet. If you eat just avoid meat, try using whey protein, eggs, non-fat cottage cheese and plain yogurt (sweetened with Stevia, if you like) as your protein choices. If you can, add fish, also.

How can a vegan use the HCG to lose weight?

This program is very difficult for a vegan. You need all 8 essential amino acids to build and repair tissue in the body. Although there are proteins and amino acids in non-animal food, they are not complete and the body does not always have what it needs to make healthy muscles and tissue. Soy is a poor substitute, as it is highly processed, most often genetically modified, and tends to suppress the thyroid, the very gland you need for better metabolism.

Also, you must take supplemental B12 as a vegan, as this vital B vitamin does not exist outside the animal world.

You can try using Quorn and some vegans have tried using tofu. Seitan is a better choice, as it is fermented soy.

I wanted to make sure the meds I'm on won't interfere. I take 50mg Cytomel for thyroid issues, Wellbutrin and Pristiq for depression, and Ortho Tri-Cyclen birth control.

Yes, you may take your meds on the FAT FIX DIET and with the Magic Drops Homeopathic HCG. In my years of clinical practice I have helped many people come off their depression medications by balancing their thyroid, which prescription medications often do not do. Iodine and natural thyroid support will help your thyroid medication to work better. Check the Thyroid symptoms and see if you need more thyroid help. Even if your blood work comes back in "normal" range, you may need additional thyroid support to get your thyroid functioning well enough to prevent depression and balance the rest of your endocrine system. Also, more thyroid support will help boost your metabolism so that you lose weight more easily.

With the fruit and Melba toast snack, does this mean I am only eating one fruit and Melba toast snack per day? What if I have a protein shake with a handful of strawberries for breakfast, does that mean I can't eat fruit for the rest of the day?

You may eat two snacks of fruit and Melba toast (skinny bread stick) per day. You may also add fruit to your protein shake in the morning, for a total of 3 fruit servings per day.

Aren't the HCG Injections stronger and better?

There are different opinions on this. I have heard many people who tried both say that they did not see much difference between the two types of HCG. Others felt that the shots were stronger and controlled their appetite better. If you have a great deal of weight to lose, 100 plus pounds, the injections may be a better choice for you. However, if you do not want to give yourself shots, or you want the safety of homeopathy, the Magic Drops work very well. There is also homeopathic appetite control that can be added to help curb your appetite. Also, the checklists in this book will help ensure your success.

What do you tell girls to do when they get their period on the diet? I think Dr. Simeons says stop taking HCG because the need for more food is greater, but it would still be in the system. So do you have them change anything?

On the Homeopathic HCG, there does not seem to be a need to stop the drops during a menstrual period. The homeopathic version is not "hormone replacement" as the original prescription version is. Some women do experience some weight gain of a couple of pounds right before their period. My advice is to stick to the program strictly. The weight gain rebalances after the period starts. Check the section on Thyroid symptoms if you have difficult periods. Many women find their periods are easier, with less cramping, and they have less PMS when doing the FAT FIX DIET.

People say that losing weight is no walk in the park. When I hear that I think, yeah, that's the problem.

Chris Adams

I had a baby 17 weeks ago, and I have about 30 lbs to shed. I had a c-section and my doctor has permitted me from doing vigorous workouts until 6 months post partum. This has left me with a problem... how do I shed this unwanted pregnancy weight? So my friend told me about this diet and I am interested in trying it out. I want to ask you a few questions regarding it first, questions like, have you had any woman with pregnancy weight do this? And was it successful for them? I don't know why but I feel like pregnancy weight is harder to get rid of then normal weight! Ha ha!

I wish I had been able to use this diet after my kids. I always lost all my baby weight but it took me a year. The FAT FIX DIET with the Magic Drops will make it much faster and easier for you, plus it is healthy, which is important for you after going through the pregnancy. Your hormones are trying to rebalance now, and the Homeopathic HCG should only help, which will mean not only faster weight loss, but also losing the extra inches that you have.

Can I use the Magic Drops during breast-feeding?

No, while you are nursing your baby let your body find its own metabolic state so that you have plenty of breast milk. Some women find they lose weight easily at this point, and others find that their body just won't let go and they need some extra fat to produce milk. As soon as you wean the baby, you can use the FAT FIX DIET to take off any remaining weight.

The Maintenance phase of the FAT FIX DIET is a healthy way to eat for you while you are breast-feeding. Eat plenty of good quality fat, and add Fish Oil capsules to your diet. You can get some moderate exercise. Try to avoid sugars and white flour completely. You can eat some whole grains like brown rice and oatmeal and rye, as you may need some extra calories to produce enough milk. Try adding in Brewer's Yeast if you find you need more milk.

If you experience any kind of post-partum depression, check the Thyroid checklist of symptoms. I have helped many women with depression and one for one I have found that the thyroid needed support. Once the thyroid is balanced and functioning well, the depression can lift completely. The good news is that this can happen in just a couple of weeks. Iodine supplementation can help, also.

I've been on the HCG diet for over 10 days now and lost 10 lbs. I am now out of town for business, away from my kitchen and food is being provided. Nothing is on the diet but I have to eat it. There's nothing else. Do I just stop the drops for the next few days, and then do the apples and start over when I get back? Help!

If you really cannot stick to the diet at all, then stop for a few days and start again when you have more control over what you eat. If you can do a modified version of the diet, then keep taking the drops. A modified version would be avoiding starches, bread, pasta and all sugars, but unable to avoid all fats and oils, for example. When you restart, if you only stop for a few days, don't binge, just go back on the program with the HCG drops. If you have to stop for 10 days or more, re-binge and plan to do 3-6 more weeks on the strict diet and Magic Drops.

I just received my HCG drops. Let me make sure I understand this. I take the drops in the morning, afternoon and evening and eat as much as I can for the first two days, correct?

Yes, binge well and it will prevent you from being hungry when you change to the protein, fruits and vegetables. Eat plenty of fatty foods that you might normally avoid. Fat is more important than sugar on the binge. If you really binge, you will probably be happy to stop eating rich foods and eat more simply on the next phase.

I have been stuck at the same weight for 4 days. What do I do?

It is not uncommon to stick at the same weight for a couple of days after 10 days or so of steady weight loss. Ride it out and stick to the diet. If it is just before your period, your weight may not shift again until your period stops, or even until your period is over. You can try an apple day, eating 6 apples only for 1 day, to see if that helps. Or you can try taking a teaspoon of fat or oil (butter, nut butter or olive oil) in the evening. Only do this once. If you still are not losing, use the Debug checklist.

Just wondering if we continue to take the drops during maintenance?

No, during the Maintenance you don't take any Magic Drops HCG. You may use a homeopathic Appetite Control, if needed. Be sure to follow the Maintenance diet strictly to reset your metabolism and lock in your lower weight.

Is it okay to use soy sauce?

Yes, look for "naturally brewed" in your Health Food store, if you can. But all soy sauce is okay.

Worcester sauce?

Yes.

Is it okay to keep taking my vitamins?

Look for food source vitamins, such as Standard Process™. Many commercial vitamins are not worth taking, and may do more harm than good in the long run, as they are not complete and may create other deficiencies.

The fruit list says melon is okay, but how much is a serving? I ate ½ a small cantaloupe last night. Is that okay?

Depends on how small. Generally, think of a serving of fruit as half a grapefruit, a handful of berries, or a medium apple.

Is sirloin steak okay if you remove the fat?

Yes, remove all fat.

How about ground sirloin as hamburger?

Look for hamburger which states low fat content or lean, or better yet, look for ground Buffalo, which is free range and naturally lean, as well as more flavorful than beef.

Should I take vitamins while on the diet?

I recommend whole food vitamins as a general rule. Look for Standard Process™ brand, or check the list at the back of this book. Don't take oil-based vitamins like Vitamin E or fish oil or Omega 3 supplements while taking the Magic Drops. But you may take these during Maintenance and afterwards.

I am a big believer in digestive enzymes and probiotics. Look for amylase, protease and lipase in your enzymes, to break down different kinds of food. If you feel full after eating meat, or it does not digest well, you may need betaine, also. The only probiotics shown to seed in the human gut is acidophilus.

If you have ever been prescribed antibiotics for an illness, you should consider probiotics. Multiple prescriptions of antibiotics? You definitely need to replace your gut flora with probiotics. Check your tongue. Grooves, white patches, red at tip or edges all indicate poor gut health. You need probiotics. Also, realize that lack of strong gut flora means you may well be B Vitamin deficient, which tongue diagnosis also reveals. Try adding Brewer's Yeast to your smoothie or shake. Of look for a natural B supplement like Cataplex B and/or Cataplex G from Standard Process.

Standard Process also make a nutritional shake powder with Whey Protein called *SP Complete* that you can use as your Whey shake during the program. It is all natural whole food nutrition that can be mixed with water, fruit and Stevia for a delicious healthy breakfast or meal replacement. They also make a very high quality Whey shake powder called Whey Pro Complete. Standard Process is available from practitioners only, so visit the website www.standardprocess.com to find someone in your area who carries the brand.

> *To promise not to do a thing is the surest way in the world to make a body want to go and do that very thing.*
>
> **Mark Twain**
> *The Adventures of Tom Sawyer,* 1876

I am checking in with you because although I'm still doing well on the HCG diet for 11 days, the past two days I have had constipation. I didn't have it before and was just wondering what you think.

I suggest that you try taking magnesium as a supplement. We have a powdered magnesium in the office that you can make into a drink, comes in flavors. Or you can try Smooth Move tea or a magnesium supplement from the health food store. It does happen on this diet. May mean you need a little gall bladder support. The magnesium is healthy for all the cells, not just to relax the intestine. Look for magnesium citrate or lactate forms. Sedona Labs makes a probiotic called *I Flora*, which helps many people to be more regular.

One client had good results taking a couple of prunes. Not really part of the diet, but it worked for her, and she still lost weight.

I would like to lose 10 more and would welcome any advice you have on doing that without going back to the full on HCG diet.

Follow the Maintenance very strictly. Many people continue to lose weight on the Maintenance. The loss will be slower, but it is a great diet for general health as well as weight loss. Also, you can increase your exercise to hard work out. The combination should work.

So once I am done with the Maintenance I am sure I will be at my ideal weight (want to lose est. 15-20 lbs). Will I be able to eat a normal 1800-2000 calorie diet? I already eat organic, very little dairy... but just wanted to know how real it was, with continuing my weekly yoga and eating well, to go back to a more usual lifestyle?

Here is the thing: I don't think it is all about calories. It is more about hormones. See "Good Calories, Bad Calories" by Gary Taubes for studies that have shown this to be true. So, you could eat 1800 calories of protein, fats and fresh produce and be slim. Or you could eat bagels and pastries and upset your insulin levels and gain weight.

Every person has to find their own way of eating that maintains their ideal weight, and that includes activity level. If you go back to eating exactly like you did before, you will probably gain all the weight back eventually. So, this is an opportunity to explore what is an ideal diet for your body. Add carbs and grains and sugars back in very slowly and see how you do. If you stay on top of it, and do a steak/protein day if you start to gain, you will be able to maintain your new lower weight.

I've read that if you can't handle Stevia or get it, that saccharin is OK, which would permit me the Sweet N Low. What do you know of this? Or advise?

One of the best things about this diet plan is the lack of processed and artificial foods. Stevia is an herb from a South American plant. It tastes sweet, but is not sugar. Saccharin was first produced in 1878 by Constantin Fahlberg, a chemist working on coal tar derivatives in a laboratory at Johns Hopkins University. Although it may not be as harmful as Aspartame, it is still chemical. By the way Sucralose (Splenda) is sugar bonded with chlorine. Stevia is a much better choice for the FAT FIX DIET and for everyday use.

Try the flavored liquid Stevia from Sweet Leaf. Many people like it even if they do not like the powdered Stevia. Also, some like the Truvia brand, available in many grocery stores.

I have a question about chewing gum – Pellu Dental Gum to be precise. Since it's not sweet, compared to regular gum and no artificial stuff. Is it OK?

Yes. Xylichew and Spry are other chewing gums that are okay on the Diet.

Just wanted to make sure no problem with mint in general because I also prefer peppermint tea.

Mint should be okay. Just be sure not to use mint close to the time you are taking the Magic Drops. Wait at least 15 minutes before and after using the Drops to put anything in your mouth.

What kind of protein shake can I use? Is Soy okay?

No Soy is allowed unless you are vegan and have few other protein choices. Soy has estrogenic properties that can suppress thyroid. Vegans may also use pea protein. The best shake powder to use is Whey protein, with nothing added to the mix. Whey protein is the most easily utilized in the body of all types of protein. Standard Process™ makes an excellent Whey product called Whey Pro.

Can I use Agave as a sweetener?

Agave is not allowed. Xylitol and Stevia are the only sweeteners allowed. Look for flavored liquid Stevia from Sweet Leaf. It comes in a variety of flavors from root beer to chocolate. These are not bitter and can add a lot of fun to your diet recipes.

I don't seem to be losing weight. Yesterday I ate nothing but apples until dinner, drank lots of water throughout the day, and had steak, onions, and salad for dinner. I have even worked out several of these days, and that combined with the eating plan should be causing calorie burning/weight loss without the HCG. Yet, I have taken 3-4 doses of the HCG each day.

Please don't make the mistake of applying other diets to this one. The FAT FIX DIET works very differently. It is important to follow the instructions very precisely in order to keep your blood sugar stable and low so that the Homeopathic HCG can be active in your system. Eat the meals as instructed at meal times and eat snacks. Don't work out more than moderately.

As my mom mentioned when she came in, I've been mildly constipated throughout the entire process. I tried Smooth Move tea, and I tried Miralax. Both helped a very little. Also, your card says No Hunger, but I am constantly starving. I'm really frustrated at this point, and losing faith in the HCG. Can you please advise me on what to do?

Use the Debug List. If you are not losing, and are constipated, there are underlying issues, like low function Thyroid or congested Gall Bladder. Follow the directions, and you should find that you can now lose.

I've been on the actual Phase 2 diet for 10 days now. If I reach my goal weight before the three week mark on this Phase 2, can I switch to "maintenance" any time? Or should I continue until I reach the 3-week mark.

It is better to do the program for 3 full weeks, even if you reach your goal sooner. Your body will not give up more weight if you don't need to lose more.

How much is a serving of vegetables?

There does not need to be a limit to the vegetables, as long as you do not add fat or oil. You may have 3 fruits per day. Try to find very lean hamburger or look for Buffalo burger, which is lean, free-range and very tasty.

We will stop taking the drops tonight (and start Maintenance) and Saturday start eating no carbs, no sugar. Can I have fruit though? I'm pretty worried about gaining 5 lbs back in a little time. We've been eating SO little and then we're going to add all this food, how can the weight not come back on? And if I do gain weight I'm supposed to do a steak day, but I don't eat red meat. What should I eat instead? Please offer me any advice you have about this next phase.

Yes, you may eat fruit on the Maintenance phase. You can use another form of protein, rather than steak, if you need to. There are homeopathic preparations for appetite control, if you feel you need that. See Products section.

Could you tell me if there is any danger as far as breast or ovarian cancers are concerned? A good friend of mine told me her sister was on HCG years ago and developed breast cancer. I have tried to do some research but wanted your opinion. Thanks so much. I hate to give up the HCG because it has worked for me so beautifully.

Sadly, many women have developed breast and ovarian cancer who never heard of HCG, so I don't see how any one can say the HCG caused cancer. There is no reason that it would, even in the prescription form. Homeopathic

I've been on a constant diet for the last two decades. I've lost a total of 789 pounds. By all accounts, I should be hanging from a charm bracelet.

Erma Bombeck

163

preparations are generally considered benign and safe, so there should not be any harm in taking the Homeopathic HCG. In fact, the FAT FIX DIET or Dr. Simeons diet are both more likely to prevent cancer, rather than cause it. These diets are anti-inflammatory and the lack of processed foods makes them very healthy.

I have to tell you that I'm actually really nervous about this diet. I am a healthy person, I eat well and exercise daily but since my baby was born one year ago I haven't been able to drop the weight. I am going to try really hard to do this but I may need some support from you in the process. For example, my in-laws are coming to town next week and they love to go to restaurants. How can I do this diet at a restaurant? And what if I slip up? I friend of mine is visiting me in 2 weeks and I can't just eat one little bland meal with her while she's here, she's a foodie (as am I) and will want to go to all the best restaurants! And what about wine? I need some wine from time to time, I know it's unrealistic to go a whole 3 weeks without a glass of wine here or there. So you see, I'm nervous about all this! Please offer me any advice you have on making this diet work through visitors and special occasions.

The best time to do the FAT FIX DIET is when you can clear your calendar for a few weeks so that you have few distractions and have a fighting chance at success. However, if your calendar never seems to clear, plunge ahead. Many people find that, if they follow the Diet and take the Homeopathic HCG strictly for at least a week, they are so pleased with the results that they are able to modify their diet much more easily during social occasions that offer a lot of temptation.

I am 30, in shape and very active, but have been struggling with the last 15-20 lbs for about 4 years now. I do a crazy diet...lose, then gain back and have been hovering around the same weight for a while, because I don't want to put my body through that again. The weight becomes harder and harder to lose. Would this diet be good for me?

This diet maybe the answer you have been looking for. Many people find they can lose weight and keep it off, despite earlier disappointments.

I have lost inches but not that much weight.

Yes, this does seem to happen with some. And some who lose many pounds the first time lose more inches than pounds the second time. As long as your clothes are fitting better and you feel good, continue the program and see what happens. You can also check the Thyroid and Adrenal checklists to see if you have symptoms that may benefit from some supplemental help.

I realized in re-reading the instructions that I have been incorrectly eating both of my fruits before I go to bed for the last week. I am also wondering whether using cocoanut oil as a vaginal lubricant would be part of the problem (½–1 tsp). I have stopped both of the above but have not noticed any difference in weight loss. I am taking Beta Food and drinking about 2L per day of alkaline water (Kangen).

Using any oil as a lubricant or moisturizer is not a good idea while taking the Magic Drops. And it is better to eat all food before 8 p.m., if possible, and only one piece of fruit at a time. I do not advise drinking Kangen or any alkaline water. Alkaline water has been used medicinally for short periods of time, but it is not true that every one is too "acid". The stomach must be very acid in order to digest protein, so acid that you could digest your fingers if you stuck your hand down your throat! The blood must be neutral at 7.2-7.4 pH. Change that and you die. So, trust your body and let Nature handle the pH of the body. Eating according to the FAT FIX DIET, eliminating grains and sugar, will help your body find its own natural balance.

My youngest daughter has a day off and we are planning a trip to Orlando—Discovery Cove park. I know this is going to be a cheat day for me, inevitably, do you have any tips? Should I take or not take the drops this day? Should I buy and take a fat/carb blocker? Any data you have on this would be invaluable. I certainly don't expect to lose any weight but I was curious what the least damaging route would be.

Even if you know that you will be breaking the diet, continue to take the drops and just continue the FAT FIX DIET as soon as you can. You may find that the drops will help curb your appetite and you will eat less junk and goodies than you expected.

No, I don't advise using carb blockers. Try to eat some Cinnamon or take some chromium to help balance your blood sugar. Also, try to eat sugar only after eating some protein and/or fat, to slow the absorption of sugar into the blood.

I have taken all of the supplements and drops you recommended and I have not deviated from the diet except I had 3½ glasses of wine one day and paid the price the next day with the runs. I have been trying to keep my exercise lighter.

If you deviate from the diet one day, know that you may experience a gain and do all you can to return to the regimen the following day. Alcohol breaks down to sugar, so it will stop the weight loss. Dr. Simeons said that ½ glass of red wine was allowed twice a week. Good idea to keep exercise light. If you exercise too heavily, you may trigger a need for more food, or upset the metabolism so that your body holds on to fat.

My mind keeps thinking I'm starving and I am starting to crave things like butter, or dressing because I am getting bored with the flavor of meat with veggies with lemon, garlic and spices so I end up using lots of salt too.

166

Check the Gall Bladder symptoms. Craving fats is a symptom of Gall Bladder congestion. Vary your protein sources between egg whites, whey protein, fish, chicken, as well as meat.

Can you drink alcohol during binge days?

I don't know of any restriction on alcohol during the binge. Please note that some people find that alcohol affects them more strongly when they are taking the Magic Drops Homeopathic HCG, so go easy!

I have osteoporosis and am taking a mixture of supplements containing one tablespoon of fish oil twice a day. Can I continue this or should I discontinue it while on the diet or reduce it to once a day?

During the phase when you are taking the Magic Drops homeopathic HCG, you should stop the fish oil. You may start the fish oil again on the Maintenance phase and I do encourage fish oil as an every day supplement for all ages. The key to bone density is not just taking calcium, but also magnesium and trace minerals, as well as making sure that you absorb calcium. Green leafy vegetables are an excellent source of calcium. Take only calcium that also contains magnesium. I like Calcium Lactate and Calcium Citrate. You can use some apple cider vinegar with your calcium supplements, as they need acid to be absorbed by the body. Try sipping some organic apple cider vinegar, 1–2 teaspoons in a cup of warm water Also, be sure to be active, as exercise is very important for bone strength.

> The commonest form of malnutrition in the western world is obesity.
>
> **Mervyn Deitel**

I have a brother who is diabetic. Type 2. He takes meds and is quite undisciplined with his diet, so as a result he is very obese. This is a simple observation from seeing how he continues to get fat and by seeing him eat BUT he is willing to be disciplined and do this diet. So my question is how should he go about it given his diabetes? I am guessing he will need supervision mostly since the 2 days of gorging he wont be able to do carbs. Do you recommend a nutritionist or someone that could supervise him? Or can he do it alone?

This is a great diet for diabetics but your brother would have to monitor his insulin closely. He will get a huge drop in blood sugar. He can gorge on fatty food, rather than on sugary foods, during the binge.

It would be best to have your brother work with a nutritionist who understands Homeopathic HCG, or a medical doctor who prescribes HCG shots. Or use one of our distributors who can help. The important thing is to monitor the blood sugar, and any other medications your brother might be taking.

I read that some people have hair loss on this diet. Is there anything I can take that can help prevent this?

I have heard this, also, but I don't see much problem with hair loss with my patients and clients. I encourage people to use the Thyroid check list and be sure to use some natural thyroid support as suggested if they have symptoms. It is almost always the thyroid that is involved with hair loss and thinning for women. By adding in some supplements, you should not have to worry about this. And there are many benefits to supporting the thyroid, in terms of assisting weight loss by boosting metabolism, improving mood and energy and helping the entire endocrine system to work better. Thyroid is very, very key to over-all health.

Also I normally take Dr. Schultz formula 1 every night to keep me regular. I didn't know if it was OK to take? Or if I needed to stick to taking what they recommend which is the "Smooth Move" tea?

I like Dr. Schulz products, but it is not ideal to take herbal stimulation to have a bowel movement every day. Check the section on Thyroid, as constipation is a symptom of functional low thyroid. Also, check Gall Bladder symptoms.

The bowel gets signals from the gall bladder and gall bladder congestion may be a reason that the intestine is sluggish. Be sure you are drinking enough water. Magnesium Lactate or Citrate may help. Moderate exercise such as walking, as well as yoga and Pilates are important. A sedentary lifestyle may be another reason for constipation.

I am considering the HCG diet but use progesterone cream daily to minimize hot flashes. I am using 1/8 tsp. twice daily of Natural Woman progesterone cream. Will I have to stop using this to do the diet?

No, most women do fine continuing with Hormone replacement during the FAT FIX DIET.

We just want to know if HCG is ineffective because she has to take Armour Thyroid.

No, the FAT FIX DIET and Magic Drops HCG will work fine for someone using Thyroid medications. I often give natural thyroid support to help the medications work better. You can use the Thyroid list to see if there are still symptoms of thyroid problems. People often need iodine supplementation, also. The Thyroid needs iodine to make Thyroxine, the main thyroid hormone. Iodine is also protective of breast and prostate cancer and helps the immune system. Iodized salt is not sufficient for many people. I like Lugol's iodine, or Iodomere. Start any iodine supplementation very slowly and increase slowly.

How many calories should I eat during the Maintenance?

Dr. Simeons suggested 1500 calories during the Maintenance. On the FAT FIX DIET, it is not how many calories, but what you eat, that counts. You can add in more protein, and more fruit. The most important change on the Maintenance Phase is to add in good quality fats. Use real organic butter and virgin olive oil. Take some Fish Oil capsules or liquid; take Evening

Primrose Oil or Flax Oil. Your skin will probably welcome the oils and your Gall Bladder functions as a response to dietary fat. Don't stop eating good fats just because you avoided fats on the HCG diet and lost weight. Fats and oils are made up of Essential fatty acids. They are called "essential" because your body must have fat to operate and the cells need fat for protection. The brain and nerve cells have a fat membrane around them. So, don't get used to a no-fat diet. Only eat low or no fat while you are taking the HCG.

You may add back in a few nuts and some dairy products. I suggest that you only use organic dairy products. See the Chapter "Happily Ever After" for a more complete explanation.

Many people find they have little appetite after the Diet Phase. Don't force it, but do add back in some good fat and increase your calories on a gradient.

The important thing is to avoid all sugars, grains, breads, pastas and starches like potatoes and beans on the Maintenance. This will reset your metabolism and ensure that you maintain your new shape and weight.

How much time should I wait before starting another round? Do I binge again?

It is a good idea to wait until after a full Maintenance to start another round of HCG. Do the full three weeks Maintenance, binge again just like before, and follow the FAT FIX DIET plan. For further rounds, try waiting 4-6 weeks between rounds. Your body needs some dietary fat and your metabolism needs to set without the Homeopathic drops. Dr. Simeons recommended waiting the same number of weeks as you used the prescription HCG because of the possibility of becoming immune to the injections. This is not such a concern with

Homeopathic HCG, but there are other good reasons to wait between rounds.

Stay on the Maintenance phase as strictly as you can during the entire period of weight loss. If you need to lose 60 pounds and you will do 3 rounds of HCG, stay on the Maintenance all the time you are not taking the Magic Drops.

Do I need to stick to the calorie restriction so tightly?

The more weight you have to lose and the more motivated you are, the more strict you should be. My advice is to be very strict for the first week or two and see how it goes and how you feel. Once you see how the diet works, and how much weight you can lose, it is easier to follow the diet strictly.

Can I eat Brussels Sprouts?

On the FAT FIX DIET you can eat any vegetable except the starchy kind like winter squash, yams and sweet potatoes, potatoes of any kind, and peas.

Can I eat anything on the binge days?

The purpose of the binge days is to get fat circulating in your system. This seems to trigger the release of fat from fat tissue, and it prevents hunger when you drop down to the actual diet of protein, vegetables and fruit. Eat fatty foods on the binge days. It is okay if the foods contain sugar, but they should also contain fat, like donuts and ice cream. Good choices are avocados, cheeseburgers, French fries, pizza, etc.

What do I do if I feel tired?

Check your water intake and salt and potassium, as you may need more. Check that you are not over-exercising and that you are getting enough sleep. The Debug checklist may be used if the problem does not clear up quickly.

> If you have formed the habit of checking on every new diet that comes along, you will find that, mercifully, they all blur together, leaving you with only one definite piece of information: french-fried potatoes are out.
>
> **Jean Kerr**

I am constipated. What do I do?

Constipation does happen with the HCG. You are eating less food, and the diet may be a big change from the usual diet for some people. Make sure you are drinking enough water. Use the Debug checklist, as this may be a thyroid or gall bladder issue. If you normally have to take something in order to eliminate, I suggest that you use gall bladder support before and during the FAT FIX DIET.

You may use magnesium to help, but look for good quality magnesium such as citrate or lactate, or use magnesium as a powdered drink. There are reports that prunes helps, but generally speaking dried fruit is not allowed, so this could slow your weight loss.

Epsom Salts (Magnesium sulphate) may be used sparingly. Try using 1-2 teaspoons in an 8 oz. glass of warm water, flavored with some fresh lemon juice. You may also soak in a tub with Epsom Salts dissolved in the water. Try 2-4 cups. Some of the magnesium will be absorbed through the skin and this is good for the body. Many enzymes require magnesium and the sulphate is good for liver function. By the way, Epsom Salts is said to help acne on face or body, when used as a soak or added to a cleansing product as a scrub.

You may also drink Ginger Tea.

I have been waking up with leg cramps. Is this from the Homeopathic HCG?

No, the drops will not cause cramps. You may be peeing out more water than usual. Be sure that you are getting enough salt, especially in hot or humid weather. Use sea salt on your food to taste. When people eliminate fast food and processed or snack foods the salt in their diet may be drastically reduced. Salt is vital for cellular function, so salt may be added to season your foods on the FAT FIX DIET. You may try adding in some magnesium and/or potassium. Also, Vitamin E supplements may help. I like Wheat Germ Oil for Vitamin E, as it is natural E, and not synthetic.

Is this diet really safe?

I would not recommend anything unless I thought it was very safe. So many people have had improved health after this program that it may be unsafe NOT to do it. The diet itself is very healthy and the Magic Drops are safe for almost anyone to take because they are homeopathic.

Can I have beans or hummus on the Maintenance?

No, avoid beans and hummus because of the high starch content while doing the Maintenance.

Why is turkey not on the list (being a lean meat) but beef is and it's a fatty meat?

Dr. Simeons' original diet did not include turkey. Many people do eat turkey on the FAT FIX DIET and do lose weight. So, if you like turkey, you can try it, but if you reach a plateau and are not losing, drop turkey out and see if that makes a difference. Beef should be as lean as possible, by the way.

Also, why can't we drink more than 64 ounces a day?

Some people may be able to drink more, but others can't seem to process that much water and it stalls their loss. If you are thirsty, drink more water. Everyone needs to drink quite a bit of water. When fat is broken down, toxins are released that were stored in the fat tissue, so it is important to drink enough water. If the weather is hot and/or humid, you may need more than 64 oz. Don't forget that you may also need salt and potassium if it is hot and you are peeing a lot. Try adding sea salt to your food and taking some potassium supplements.

How to order from you, give credit card number? Send check?

You can give a credit card by phone or fax to (206) 202 4499, or order online at www.annedunev.com.

You may also order from the Distributors listed in their section. All of the distributors are trained in the FAT FIX DIET using the Magic Drops Homeopathic HCG and they are eager to help you achieve your weight loss goals.

The Key to Enjoying
the Food on the Diet

This is a time to explore seasonings, spices and extra tools for cooking. You can use a variety of ethnic seasonings to flavor your food. Asian, Mexican, Italian and Indian are a few of the choices you have so that you aren't facing a poached, bland chicken breast. You can cook ahead and freeze individual portions to take with you, or grab when you are hungry.

Lemon juice, garlic, curry, Tabasco, chili peppers and soy sauce can all be used, along with fresh and dried herbs. Great flavor will go far in helping you to satisfy your appetite on lower calories. And you may find natural flavors far superior to the chemical artificial flavors that are cheap substitutes for the genuine thing. In the U.S. we have almost forgotten that Nature made flavors first. So, this diet can be gourmet, if you can get creative.

If you don't cook much, you will have to hunt down food that does not have the fake oils, chemicals and sugar that almost all prepared and packaged foods contain. Try your local health food store. Frozen food is allowed, but fresh is always better. Canned foods may contain extra salt or sugar, so read the label.

Nothing tastes as good as being thin feels.

Author Unknown

175

If you have a friend who cooks who would like to do the diet, you may be able to work out some exchange if he/she will cook your portions and fill your freezer.

It is vital to organize the food ahead of time so that you are not starving and searching for the first edible thing to stuff in your mouth. Keep veggies and fruit close by, and organize your protein choices so that you are always prepared with the right food when you need it.

If you have been relying on fast food and drive-through, you could be shocked at how good you feel eating real food for a change. Most people feel very good on this diet, and cannot go back to their previous life-style.

In the Recipe section you will find suggested tools to help you cook fast and delicious entrees.

Eating So You Can Stick to the Diet

A few people are able to eat plain chicken and one vegetable, or fish and a vegetable, for every meal and the bread stick and apple as a snack day in and day out and lose weight on the HCG eating plan.

But most of us get bored with plain food and need to mix it up a bit. Fortunately, there are many condiments, spices and seasonings allowed, so you can actually prepare "gourmet" HCG recipes.

You will also be able to eat out and still lose weight.

The secret is in the organization. It is better that you enjoy the food and feel that you are eating well, instead of dieting and depriving yourself. And, if you are cooking for family members, it is helpful if you can make recipes that others can enjoy with you. Just remember that children and adults not on the diet need dietary fat. More about that in the "Truth About Fats" section.

You don't want to arrive home from work starving, with nothing ready to eat except a box of crackers and a pint of ice cream.

There are a few tricks that work very well, if you have some tools and plan ahead.

Equipment for the Kitchen

Counter-top grill

One piece of equipment I highly recommend is a George Foreman Grill. This is the counter-top version and a small one costs only about $30. In just 5-6 minutes you can have a delicious grilled piece of steak, chicken or fish. The fat will drain into a small trough, leaving the meat or fish juicy and flavorful. You can add garlic, lemon, salt and pepper or other spices during grilling, or afterwards. You can even grill vegetables. This is food that you and your family will enjoy that is healthy and delicious.

Outdoor Grill

Of course, there is nothing like the smell of barbecued meat or chicken. The challenge to outdoor grilling is the difficulty of avoiding fat to keep things from sticking. You can use one of the vegetable oil sprays, or wrap food in aluminum foil. You can also use a grill pan instead of grilling directly on the rack. Make your own oil-free barbecue sauce.

Crock Pot

I use a crock pot often as a working Mom. You can prepare food the night before, if mornings are stressful. Refrigerate and put it all together in the crock pot before you leave for work. Arrive home to delicious aromas and a ready meal. Pasta sauce, chili and stews and chicken dishes, can all be made in a crock-pot.

Veggie Pasta Machine

A zucchini/vegetable cutting machine allows you to make zucchini "pasta". Feed the zucchini in one end, turn the handle, and out comes long "strings" from the other end. On Phase II of the diet you can prepare a simple tomato-based pasta sauce that is delicious over the steamed or boiled zucchini. Add some ground buffalo or well-drained lean cooked hamburger or cooked shrimp or diced chicken and you have a complete meal. For your family you can add a bit of olive oil and grated cheese. Your children may enjoy the zucchini pasta as a great substitute, or you can cook wheat, rice or other pasta for them.

Grater

Make veggie rice by lightly steaming grated cauliflower to mimic rice.

The Healthiest Foods
You Can Eat

This list was compiled by Dr. Weston A. Price. Dr. Price traveled around the world in the 1930s and 40s to study the health of people eating their native/traditional diets, and what happened when refined white flour and sugar was added. His book, called "Diet and Physical Degeneration" is a bible among traditional Nutritionists who recommend whole food diets for anti-aging and avoiding chronic disease. See www.westonaprice.org for more information.

- Butter from grass-fed cows (preferably organic raw butter)

- Oysters

- Liver from grass-fed animals

- Eggs from organic free-range hens

- Cod liver oil

- Fish eggs

- Whole raw milk from grass-fed cows

- Bone broth (see Weston Price website for information on preparation)

- Wild salmon

Rich, fatty foods are like destiny: they too, shape our ends.

Author Unknown

- Whole organic yoghurt or kefir

- Beef from grass-fed steers

- Sauerkraut

- Organic Beets

These foods provide concentrated nutrients needed for cellular health. The cells of the brain and nervous system have a sheath around them, composed of 80% fat and 20% protein. This protects the cell, and allows the transmission of nerve impulses, and a path for regeneration in case of injury. Loss of this sheath is a marker of many degenerative diseases. So, eating the right kind and amount of healthy fats and protein are protective of these cells.

Heart disease barely existed before 1900, when we ate lard (animal fat), real butter, and plenty of animal protein. Margarine requires the use of metals such as aluminum and nickel in order to make the vegetable oil solid in a process called "hydrogenation". Many other chemicals and flavor enhancers are added. This is not a "natural" food!

> *Let your food be your medicine and your medicine be your food.*
>
> HIPPOCRATES 460 BC

What is "junk" food? Food that has little or no nutritional value. If you want to be slim and healthy, 90% of the food you eat must have nutrients that repair and rebuild the cells of the body. So, skinny is not always healthier. What really determines the health of the body is how many healthy cells you have. Healthy cells withstand attacks from bacteria, viruses, fungus and toxins like chemicals and metals. The health of your cells determines your cancer risk because healthy cells reproduce healthy new cells, not mutants that form tumors.

High quality, nutrient-dense food can be delicious. Think fine French, Italian and Spanish cuisine! Your mental and physical health are both affected strongly by the foods you eat. Food is your friend, but you have to know how to find the real thing. Junk food only loves you for a few minutes, then lets you down by piling on fat and loading you with chemicals. Real food keeps your body strong and resilient and loves you all of your life.

Recipes to Inspire You

All recipes are for use on Phase 2 (no fat/low calories) unless otherwise noted. For Phase 3 (Maintenance phase), oil, butter, dairy and/or nuts may be added.

If I had been around when Rubens was painting, I would have been revered as a fabulous model. Kate Moss? Well, she would have been the paintbrush.

Dawn French

Salads and Dressings

COLESLAW

> ½ head Grated Cabbage
> Bean Sprouts (optional)
> 2 tbsp Apple Cider Vinegar
> ½ tsp powdered ginger or 1 tsp grated fresh ginger
> ½ tsp Soy Sauce   *Tamara GF*

Mix sauce and pour over cabbage. May add diced cooked chicken breast if desired to make complete meal.

SUMMER TOMATO SALAD

Baby Heirloom Tomatoes, cut in half, or Chopped Fresh Tomatoes, or Cherry Tomatoes cut in half- Use only fresh seasonal tomatoes

> 10 Leaves fresh Basil, chopped or torn into small pieces
> 1-2 tbsp Reduced Balsamic Vinegar (see recipe below)
> Sea Salt and pepper to taste.
> Toss all ingredients together.

Reduced Balsamic Vinegar
1 Bottle good quality Italian Balsamic Vinegar

Simmer in saucepan for 1 hour or until liquid is reduced to ⅓-½ of original volume. Sauce will thicken when it cools, so don't reduce too much. Watch and stir often so vinegar does not burn bottom of pan.

This brings out the sweetness of the vinegar and it can be used as a topping for cooking chicken, meat or fish. It can be used to replace all or some of vinegar in a salad dressing. It can be used alone when a sweet tasting salad dressing is desired. Delicious for grilling vegetables, too. Drizzle over vegetables before roasting or grilling.

SWEET "HONEY" MUSTARD DRESSING

½ tsp of your favorite mustard
2 to 3 tbsp reduced balsamic vinegar

Mix together to make a dressing for salad or vegetables or use over chicken or meat.

CREAMY BUTTERMILK RANCH DRESSING

This recipe is a bit of a cheat, but could be used in sparingly for a treat.

½ cup cottage cheese, low fat or non-fat
⅓ cup plain yogurt
1 clove garlic–minced
2 tablespoons chopped chives
Salt and pepper to taste

Place all the ingredients in the bowl of a food processor fitted with the steel blade. Process until smooth.

YOGURT DRESSING

>2 medium cucumbers, peeled and seeded, coarsely chopped or shredded
>¼ tsp cayenne pepper or Tabasco
>2 tsp white wine vinegar (try white balsamic)
>2 cups plain yogurt (organic)
>1 tbsp dill

Marinate cucumbers in bowl with vinegar and seasonings. Drain liquid and mix with yogurt and dill. Add Tabasco or cayenne and chill before serving. May be used as dressing or dip for fresh vegetables.

CURRIED VEGETABLE SALAD

>1 cup plain yogurt
>1 tbsp curry powder
>1 tbsp red wine or balsamic vinegar
>1 medium clove garlic, crushed
>1 tsp salt and dash of pepper
>2 cups of vegetables: sliced cucumber, zucchini, tomatoes, with cooked cubed eggplant.

Mix sauce and serve over vegetables, toss gently.

CREAMY FRENCH DRESSING

>1 cup nonfat cottage cheese, puréed
>1 tsp tomato juice
>1 tsp paprika
>1 tsp dry mustard
>1 tsp Worcestershire sauce
>1 tsp onion powder
>1 tsp garlic powder, or to taste
>Additional tomato juice to thin, if necessary

CREAMY ITALIAN DRESSING

    1 cup nonfat cottage cheese, puréed
    ½ tsp oregano
    ½ tsp garlic powder
    ½ tsp onion flakes

Stir spices in puréed cottage cheese.

CREAMY DILL DRESSING

    1 cup non fat cottage cheese
    1 tbsp lemon juice
    1 dash Sea Salt
    1 tbsp fresh dill
    1 tbsp onion, minced

Place cottage cheese, lemon juice, and salt in blender jar. Blend until creamy, adding water if needed to produce desired consistency.

Mix in chopped fresh dill and minced onion. Chill.

LEMON DRESSING

    ½ lemon, peeled.
    ⅛ tsp Stevia

Blend in blender or small "bullet" blender or food processor until smooth. Add water to desired consistency. Use on salad, grilled vegetables, or fruit. Also may be used on chicken.

CHICKEN STRAWBERRY SPINACH SALAD

    3.5 oz. chicken breast, diced
    ½ tsp garlic powder
    ½ lime, juiced
    ½ tsp ground ginger
    2 cups fresh spinach, stems removed

4-6 fresh strawberries, sliced
1 grissini bread stick, crumbled
Sea salt
Freshly ground black pepper to taste

Heat chicken in skillet, season with garlic powder and cook 10 minutes on medium on each side or until juices run clear. Set aside. In a bowl, mix lime juice and ginger. Arrange spinach on serving dishes. Top with chicken and strawberries, sprinkle with crumbled bread stick and drizzle with dressing. Season with pepper and serve.

Tomato Salad

Chopped tomato
Green onion
Cilantro
Jalapeno
Sea salt
Freshly ground black pepper

Add lemon if desired. You have to taste it and occasionally add more tomato to cut the spiciness, or add more jalapeno.

Creole Chicken Salad

Chicken
Cajun seasoning
Lettuce
Yellow onion
Tomatoes
Sea salt
Freshly ground black pepper

Completely coat chicken breast with Cajun seasoning and grill. Slice and serve over salad, sprinkle with salt, pepper, and lemon juice if desired.

> My doctor told me to stop having intimate dinners for four. Unless there are three other people.
> **Orson Welles**

Chicken Salad (or Crab salad, if you're eating seafood)

3 to 6 oz chicken or crab (real crab only)
7 oz celery
Herbs
Sea salt
Freshly ground black pepper

Dice chicken or crab very fine. Chop celery. Add dash of mustard, salt, pepper, cayenne, vinegar, and whatever herbs you like (savory and parsley work well). Mix all the ingredients together in a bowl.

Served chilled.

Strawberry Vinaigrette Dressing

Strawberries
½ tsp apple cider vinegar
1 tsp lemon juice
Stevia to taste
Dash salt
Dash cayenne
Freshly ground black pepper to taste

Combine all ingredients in food processor. Purée until smooth. Pour over fresh arugala or green salad. Garnish with sliced strawberries and freshly ground pepper. Variation: use as a marinade or sauce. Makes 1 serving (1 fruit)

Shrimp Salad

Marinate shrimp overnight in Old Bay seasoning and a splash of lime juice. Grill and serve over salad.

OLD BAY SHRIMP

> ½ cup cider vinegar
> ½ cup water
> 2 tablespoons OLD BAY® Seasoning

Bring to boil over medium heat.

Add 1 pound large shrimp, peeled and deveined, leaving tails on. Steam until shrimp is cooked through. Serve with cocktail sauce. Page 114

STEAK SALAD

> Steak
> Lettuce OR Spinach OR Red Onion OR Radishes
> OR Red Cabbage
> Tomato
> Sea Salt
> Freshly Ground Black Pepper

Grill steak until medium. Slice very thin. Chop vegetable of choice and serve room temperature, steak over salad. Season with salt and pepper.

SPINACH AND MEAT SALAD

> Baby Spinach
> Chicken Breasts or Beef, grilled and chopped
> Strawberries, sliced
> ¼ cup Apple Cider Vinegar
> 2-3 packets Stevia
> Sea Salt
> Freshly Ground Black Pepper

Place clean spinach in a large salad bowl. Top with beef or chicken and strawberries. Mix vinegar with Stevia and pour over salad.

CHICKEN AND SALAD

> Chicken Breast, diced
> Garlic
> Oregano
> Sea Salt
> Freshly Ground Black Pepper

Place clean spinach in a large salad bowl. Top with beef or chicken and strawberries. Mix vinegar with Stevia and pour over salad.

WALDORF SALAD

> Lots of Celery, diced
> 1 Apple, diced
> Chicken, cooked in cider vinegar and spices and diced
> Juice of one or two Lemon wedges
> 1 or 2 tbsp Apple Cider Vinegar
> 1 or 2 packets of Stevia
> Cinnamon

Mix all together. Variation: Greens, Oranges, and Beef, with Orange flavored Stevia instead of the cinnamon.

ONION SALAD DRESSING

> 1 tbsp chopped onion
> ¼ lemon, juiced
> ¼ tsp basil
> ¼ tsp oregano
> ¼ tsp cumin
> Sea salt to taste
> Freshly ground black pepper to taste

Combine all ingredients and shake until blended.

ZESTY SALAD DRESSING

> Juice of ½ lemon
> Apple cider vinegar (or vinegar of choice)
> ⅛ teaspoon of dried mustard
> Garlic, pepper, paprika, oregano and other seasoning to taste.

Put all ingredients in a container, cover and shake until blended.

CHICKEN SALAD

Season serving of chicken breast with allowed spices, grill and slice. Serve over green leaf lettuce, butter lettuce or spinach. Add Zesty Salad Dressing.

> More die in the United States of too much food than of too little.
>
> **John Kenneth Galbraith**
> *The Affluent Society*

Marinades and Sauces

SPICY MARINADE

> 1 tsp red chili pepper flakes or 3 chopped jalapenos
> 10 green onions, chopped
> ½ cup chopped onion
> 4 garlic cloves, chopped
> 4 bay leaves, crushed
> 1 three inch piece ginger, peeled and chopped or 1 tbsp dried ginger
> ⅓ cup fresh thyme or 2 tbsp dried thyme
> 1 teaspoon freshly ground nutmeg or dried nutmeg
> 1 teaspoon freshly ground cinnamon or dried cinnamon
> 1 tablespoon freshly ground black pepper
> ¼ cup lime juice

Mix ingredients together and refrigerate to use as marinade

Cocktail Sauce

  1 cup sugar-free tomato sauce

  1 tsp onion powder

  ½ tsp celery salt

  ¼ tsp paprika

  2 tsp fresh chopped parsley

  1 tsp stevia

  1 tsp worcestershire sauce

  1 tsp fresh lemon juice

  2 tsp drained, prepared horseradish

  ½ tsp hot sauce

  Cumin to taste

  Sea salt

  Freshly ground black pepper

Combine all ingredients and serve with chilled, cooked shrimp.

Homemade BBQ Sauce

  1 small onion, minced

  1 clove garlic, minced or ½ tsp garlic powder

  1 can (6oz) tomato paste

  Stevia to taste

  ¼ cup sugar free ketchup

  3 tsp mustard

  1 tsp worcestershire sauce

  Hot sauce to taste

  ½ cup water

  Bragg liquid amino acids

Pan-fry the onion in broth or Bragg's Amino Acids over medium heat until tender. Add garlic clove and stir. Add the remaining ingredients, including water. Stir. Allow to simmer for 20-30 minutes. Stevia will tone down the spiciness if needed.

SALSA

    Ripe, fresh tomatoes
    Cilantro
    Cayenne
    Lemon juice
    Apple cider vinegar
    Sea salt

Blend the tomatoes and add spices.

MARINARA SAUCE

    1 medium onion
    2 cloves garlic, peeled and chopped or 2 tsp.
    Chopped garlic from jar
    2 cans Italian peeled tomatoes
    1 tsp. Oregano
    1 tsp chopped parsley, fresh or dried (optional)
    Few flakes red pepper flakes
    Salt to taste

Sauté onion in water or beef broth. Add garlic, oregano, parsley, red pepper flakes. Add tomatoes and cook over medium heat until sauce is simmering. Add salt to taste. Lower heat and continue to cook sauce until tomatoes are soft.

As sauce cooks, tomatoes may be broken up with spoon. Adjust seasonings. For a less chunky sauce, blend until smooth.

Sauce may be cooked in crock pot, after onion and garlic and spices are cooked and tomatoes are added. Cook on low for several hours or high for 3 hours.

Sauce may be used over grilled chicken, or cooked vegetables.

Cooked ground buffalo or low fat organic ground beef may be added.

MARINADE FOR MEAT

     1 cup tomato juice, sauce or purée

     ½ cup tomato juice and red wine

     1 minced clove garlic

     ½ tsp each marjoram and thyme

     1 large shredded onion

     2 tbsp Worcestershire sauce

     ¼ tsp freshly ground black pepper

     2 tbsp chopped parsley

Cut meat into serving sizes, put into marinade, and soak 2-3 hours or refrigerate overnight.

TOMATO VINAIGRETTE FOR USE ON MEATS

     ½ cup chopped tomatoes

     2 tbsp balsamic vinegar

     ½ tsp dried or fresh basil

     ½ tsp ground mustard

In a blender or small food processor, blend of process the tomatoes, vinegar, basil, thyme, and mustard on medium to high speed, about 25 seconds. Store in refrigerator. Shake well before serving.

Soups

TOMATO BASIL SOUP

> 3 large ripe Tomatoes, peeled and chopped, or one 16 oz large can of fire roasted tomatoes
> 1 Onion, peeled and finely chopped
> 1 clove Garlic, crushed
> Fresh Basil Leaves
> 1 cup Fat-Free Chicken or Vegetable Stock
> 1 tbsp Tomato Purée
> Sea Salt
> Freshly Ground Black Pepper to taste

Stir in 1 serving (3 to 6 oz. chicken) to make it a main dish. If prepared with vegetable stock, it will be suitable for vegetarians.

Forget love – I'd rather fall in chocolate!
Attributed to Sandra J. Dykes

FRENCH ONION SOUP

> 2 cans Fat-Free Chicken Stock
> 1 Beef Bouillon Cube
> 1 dash Worcestershire Sauce
> 2 medium Onions, sliced thin
> 2 packets Stevia
> Sea Salt
> Freshly Ground Black Pepper to taste

Stir fry the onions with a little of the chicken stock, salt, and pepper until soft/browned. Bring the rest of the ingredients to a boil in separate pot, then add the onions and let simmer for about 20 minutes.

SHRIMP GUMBO

> 3 to 6 oz Shrimp
> 7 oz (or more) chopped Celery

Dash of Cayenne Pepper
Sea Salt
Freshly Ground Black Pepper

Put everything in a saucepan with a dash of Apple Cider Vinegar and cover until the celery is slightly cooked and shrimp are fully cooked.

CHICKEN CELERY SOUP

Chicken breast
Celery
2 tbsp Minced onion, dried
Italian seasoning
Pinch cayenne
Salt and pepper
Garlic if desired

Use water to cover. Simmer all together. Use at least one stalk of celery for each 3.5 ounces of meat.

GAZPACHO

4 ripe tomatoes, quartered
1 small onion, coarsely chopped
1 peeled garlic clove
½ cup water
2 tablespoons lemon juice
Pepper to taste
Cayenne (optional)
1 sprig fresh parsley
4 ice cubes
1 medium cucumber, peeled and coarsely chopped

Blend all ingredients in a blender or food processor.

ZUCCHINI SOUP

¼ Cup diced onion
1 cup thinly sliced carrots
1 cup thinly sliced zucchini
2 teaspoons chopped fresh parsley
¼ tsp thyme
⅛ teaspoon pepper
2 cups water

In a 1 ½ quart saucepan, cook onion until translucent; add all other ingredients except water. Cover and cook over low heat, stirring occasionally, until vegetables are tender, about 10 minutes. Add water and bring to a boil. Reduce heat to medium and cook until vegetables are soft, about 20 minutes. Remove from heat and let cool slightly. Remove ½ cup soup from pan and reserve; pour remaining soup into blender and process at low speed until smooth. Combine puréed and reserved mixtures in saucepan and cook, stirring constantly until hot. Makes two servings.

LEMON CHICKEN SOUP (DEANNA)

3.5 to 5 oz. Chicken breast, diced
2 ½ to 3 cups water
Garlic, salt, pepper, paprika, and other seasonings to taste
Serving of asparagus
Juice of ½ lemon
Fresh cilantro diced

Cook chicken and seasonings in water until done. Add asparagus and cook 3 to 4 more minutes. Squeeze lemon half into soup, add cilantro and serve.

Main Dishes

SEAFARER WRAP UPS

>   1 large head iceberg lettuce
>   ½ tsp salt
>   16 oz haddock or other white fish fillets
>   4 tbsp lemon juice
>   1 cup diced fresh mushrooms
>   ½ cup finely chopped green onions
>   1 tbsp chopped parsley
>   1 tsp fennel seed
>   ⅛ tsp pepper
>   1 clove garlic, crushed

Remove core from lettuce. Carefully remove 8 outer leaves. Save remaining lettuce for salad.

In a large saucepan heat 1-1/2 quarts water and ¼ tsp salt to boiling. Add outer lettuce leaves and cook for 1 minute, until soft and pliable. Rinse under cold water and drain on paper towels.

Cut fish into 8 pieces. In small bowl combine lemon juice with remaining ingredients. Place a piece of fish on each lettuce leaf. Spoon 2 TBLS of filling on top of each. Fold in sides of leaves and roll up jelly roll style to form a tight bundle. Place each bundle on a broiler pan and broil 4 inches from heat 9-12 minutes or until fish flakes with fork. Makes 4 servings.

MOROCCAN KABOBS

>   1 lb boneless beef tenderloin steaks, cut 1 inch thick

MARINADE:

>   ⅛ cup Stevia

3 tbsp orange juice

2 cloves garlic, minced

¼ tsp ground cumin

Cut beef steak into 1-1/4 inch pieces. Whisk marinade ingredients in large bowl until smooth. Add beef; toss to coat. Cover and marinate in refrigerator 30 minutes to 2 hours.

Soak eight 6-inch bamboo skewers in water 10 minutes; drain. Remove beef from marinade; discard marinade. Thread beef pieces onto skewers, leaving small space between pieces.

Place kabobs on grid over medium, ash-covered coals. Grill, uncovered, 6 to 8 minutes (over medium heat on preheated gas grill, covered, 7 to 9 minutes) for medium rare (145°F) to medium (160°F) doneness, turning occasionally.

I have gained and lost the same ten pounds so many times over and over again my cellulite must have déjà vu.

Jane Wagner

HALIBUT WITH CUCUMBERS AND DILL

(From New York Times—Martha Rose Shulman)

   2 medium cucumbers, peeled if waxed, or 1 European seedless cucumber

   3 tablespoons chopped fresh dill

   Salt and freshly ground pepper

   1 ½ lbs halibut fillets

   2 large garlic cloves, minced

   1 or 2 shallots, minced (optional)

   ¼ cup fresh lemon juice

   1 tbsp extra virgin olive oil—omit for Main Diet program, but okay for Maintenance phase

   ¼ cup dry white wine

Preheat the oven to 425 degrees. If using regular cucumbers, cut in half lengthwise, scoop out the seeds and slice thin. If using a European cucumber, just slice thin. Oil a baking dish large enough to accommodate the fish fillets in one layer. Cut

199

a piece of parchment the size of the baking dish, and set it aside. Line the baking dish with half of the cucumber slices. Sprinkle on 1 tablespoon of the dill and salt and pepper lightly.

Rinse the fish fillets, and pat dry. With the tip of a sharp knife, score them on the diagonal a few times (this prevents them from curling when they cook). Lay on top of the cucumbers. Salt and pepper lightly, and sprinkle on the garlic and shallot. Sprinkle with another tablespoon of the dill, and drizzle on half the lemon juice and the olive oil. Top with the remaining cucumbers. Add the remaining lemon juice, and sprinkle the remaining dill over the top layer of cucumbers. Add the white wine, and cover with the parchment. Cover the dish tightly with foil, and place in the oven. Bake 10 to 15 minutes until the fish is opaque and pulls apart when stuck with a fork.

Remove from the oven, let sit for a few minutes and then serve from the baking dish, spooning some of the liquid from the baking dish over the top.

Yield: Serves four.

ADVANCE PREPARATION: If you wish, you can assemble the dish ahead of time, but don't add the lemon juice or wine. Cover with plastic, and refrigerate for one hour or longer. When ready to bake, add the lemon juice and wine.

SPANISH OMELET
    3 Egg Whites
    1 Whole Egg
    Cumin
    Onion, diced
    Tomato, diced
    Sea Salt to taste
    Freshly Ground Black Pepper to taste

Use different herbs and/or veggie to change this up. Tomato counts as fruit.

Lunch or Dinner "Wraps"

BUFFALO SLIDERS

>   6 oz. Ground buffalo
>   Iceberg lettuce, washed and left in large leaves
>   Sugar free ketchup, hot sauce, salsa, mustard, other condiments go taste

Shape the ground buffalo into 3 "fingers" or oblong patties. Grill or sauté until rare or medium rare.

Arrange on a large lettuce leaf, with sauce or condiments, wrap lettuce around and enjoy.

ORGANIC BEEF SLIDERS

Look for organic ground beef, 98% fat free. Prepare as above.

TACO LETTUCE WRAPS

>   6 oz. Lean ground beef or ground buffalo
>   Mix spices and set aside:
>   ¾ tsp cumin or to taste
>   ¼ tsp chili pepper or to taste
>   ¼ tsp red pepper or to taste
>   ¼ tsp oregano or to taste
>   ¼ tsp onion powder to taste
>   ¼ tsp garlic or to taste
>   Sea salt
>   Freshly ground black pepper
>   ¾ cup water
>   Iceberg or Romaine lettuce leaves

Brown meat, drain, and pat with paper towel. Place meat back in pan. Sprinkle spices on top and add water. Heat, then simmer for 15 minutes. Divide into servings and serve wrapped in lettuce leaves.

Chicken Fajita Wraps
    6 oz chicken breast, sliced into small pieces
    2 cooked, canned or 2 small fresh tomatoes
    Hot sauce to taste such as tabasco
    Hot chili pepper flakes
    Dash cumin
    Salt to taste
    ½ tsp chopped garlic
    Several leaves of washed iceberg lettuce

Cook all together in frying pan until chicken is cooked through. May need to add some water to prevent chicken from drying out, depending on juiciness of tomatoes. Arrange 2 spoons of the mixture on a lettuce leaf, wrap, and enjoy.

Steak Fajita Wraps

Same recipe as above, but use sliced steak instead. Steak may be grilled partially in a George Foreman Grill. Then transfer to frying pan with other ingredients and continue cooking until juice is absorbed. Wrap in lettuce leaves and enjoy.

Ground Meat and Vegetable Soup
    1 can tomato purée
    1-2 chopped onions
    2 chopped stalks celery
    2 diced carrots
    1 minced clove garlic
    1-2 tsp salt

1 bay leaf

Pinch of marjoram, thyme or other savory herbs

2 qts. Soup stock or fat-free stock or bouillon or vegetable cooking water

½ tsps freshly ground peppercorns

1 lb lean ground beef or ground buffalo

Combine first 8 ingredients in soup kettle. Cover pot and simmer until vegetables are almost tender, about 10 minutes. Add stock or liquid of choice from ingredients list.

Pinch meat to small bits and add, stirring rapidly.

Taste for seasoning, heat to simmering and serve. Garnish with parsley.

> To lengthen your life, shorten your meals.
>
> **Proverb**

VEGETABLE PURÉE

Liquefy in a blender, with 1 cup water or stock or vegetable cooking water, the following vegetables:

1 carrot

1 onion

Choose among the following:

Spinach, celery, celery root, tomatoes, leeks, broccoli, leeks, zucchini.

Pinch each of basil, marjoram, or other savory herbs to taste.

1 tsp Worcestershire sauce

1 tsp salt

Add vegetables to 1 cup boiling soup stock. Boil 1 minute, reduce heat, add herbs, Worcestershire and salt.

Simmer no longer than 8 minutes. Adjust seasonings and serve.

Vegetables

GRILLED ASPARAGUS

    Asparagus

    Lemon juice

    Sea salt

    Fresh ground black pepper

    Season asparagus with salt and pepper. Sprinkle with lemon juice and grill.

    Grilled Tomatoes with Garlic

    Ripe fresh tomatoes

    4 cloves garlic, minced

    Sea salt

    Fresh or dried basil

Preheat oven to 350 degrees F (175 degrees C). Slice tomatoes, and sprinkle with minced garlic and basil. Arrange tomatoes in a single layer on a baking sheet. Sprinkle with salt. Bake tomatoes about 20 minutes in the preheated oven, until slightly shriveled. Serve warm. For Phase 3 (Maintenance and Forever After) — May drizzle tomatoes with 2 T Extra Virgin Olive Oil before baking. May also broil or grill.

GRILLED ONION

    1 large onion, peeled

    Seasoned salt to taste

    Garlic powder

    Sea salt

    Freshly ground black pepper

Slice onion into rings and place onion on foil. Sprinkle with seasoned salt, salt, pepper, and garlic. Place the onion on a grill or in the oven under broiler, and cook until the onion is soft, about 20 minutes.

COLESLAW

Grated cabbage
Fresh grated ginger or powdered ginger
Rice wine vinegar
Stevia
Onion powder
Sea salt
Freshly ground black pepper

Combine the cabbage and herbs. Season with salt and pepper. Combine dressing ingredients in a small jar and shake. Combine with salad. Very refreshing. Add chopped cooked chicken for main dish.

EGGPLANT ROLL UPS ITALIANA

For the sauce:

1 8 oz can tomato sauce
½ cup jarred roasted red peppers, patted dry and chopped
2 cloves garlic, crushed
½ teaspoon dried basil
½ teaspoon dried oregano
¼ teaspoon salt
freshly ground black pepper

Combine tomato sauce, peppers, garlic, basil, oregano, and salt in a blender; add pepper to taste. Process until smooth.

For the eggplant:

2–3 large Italian eggplant, tops and bottoms trimmed
cooking spray
salt and freshly ground
black pepper

3 packed cups spinach leaves, chopped
1 ½ cups skim cottage cheese
¼ teaspoon dried basil
¼ teaspoon dried oregano

To make the eggplant rolls, position oven rack about 6 inches from heat source and preheat broiler. Place an eggplant on a cutting board so the bottom end faces you. Cut a thin slice lengthwise off two opposite sides to remove skin, then discard. Cut the rest lengthwise into 1/2-inch-thick slices. Repeat with other eggplant to make 12 slices total. Coat both sides of eggplant slices with cooking spray and season with salt and pepper.

Working in two batches, place slices on a foil-lined baking sheet and broil for 2 to 4 minutes on each side or until lightly browned. Remove from oven and set aside to cool. Turn off broiler and preheat oven to 350°F. Coat a skillet with cooking spray and place over medium heat. Add spinach. Season with salt and cook about 2 minutes or until wilted. Transfer spinach to a bowl and mix with ricotta, basil, and oregano; add pepper to taste.

Place a rounded tablespoon of cottage cheese mixture near one end of an eggplant slice and roll eggplant up. Place in a baking dish, seam side down; repeat with remaining slices. Pour sauce over rolls and bake for 20 minutes.

Serve on individual plates or family-style.

VEGETABLE PASTA

Slice zucchini into thin strips and steam or boil. Squeeze out excess water and serve with marinara sauce (with meat) for complete meal.

CARROTS WITH THYME

> 2 cups cut large or baby carrots
> 1 tsp. fresh or ½ tsp dried thyme
> ½ tsp. stevia mixed with ⅓ cup water

Place carrots in baking dish. Pour stevia/water mix over and sprinkle with Thyme. Bake at 350 until tender, about 20 minutes.

I am not a glutton—I am an explorer of food.

Erma Bombeck

ZUCCHINI, TOMATOES, APPLES & ONIONS

> 1 ½ lb small zucchini, thinly sliced
> ⅓ cup water or chicken bouillon or stock
> 1 medium onion, chopped
> 2 apples, chopped
> 2 fresh tomatoes, peeled and chopped or 2 canned tomatoes, chopped
> 2 tablespoons fresh chopped parsley
> Fresh ground black pepper to taste

Set a small pan of water to boil. Drop the zucchini slices into the boiling water for 30 seconds. Remove immediately and drain. Heat water or stock in a fry pan and sauté the onion until it is transparent. Add the apples and stir well to coat. Add the tomatoes and the blanched zucchini. Stir well, and then add the parsley. Season this mixture, and leave it to cook, covered over a gentle heat for 5-10 minutes, until the zucchini is soft. Serve hot.

CAULIFLOWER "RICE"

> 1 head fresh cauliflower with outer leaves and stem cut off
> 2 tbsp water

Grate cauliflower with food processor or hand grater. Place "rice" in a pot with water. Steam the cauliflower until it is

207

"al dente" or still firm, but cooked. Serve with a sauce, such as the Asian vinegar sauce, Curry sauce or Bolognese sauce or any other seasonings of your choice.

Fish

GRILLED WHITEFISH
> ¼ cup fresh orange juice
> 1 ½ tbsp lemon juice
> 3 tbsp lime juice
> ⅛ tsp cayenne pepper
> 2 minced garlic cloves
> 2 tbsp olive oil
> 1 lb cod filets
> 2 tbsp finely chopped fresh chives
> 1 tbsp finely chopped fresh thyme

Combine orange, lemon and lime juices in a bowl with cayenne pepper, garlic, olive oil and 1/3 cup of water to make the marinade. Place fish in a flat dish and pour in the marinade and then marinate the fish 15 minutes. Light your grill and add the fish – grill fish 3 to 4 minutes per side, basting often with the marinade. Serve the fish with a spoonful of marinade and sprinkle with chives and thyme.

SPICY SNAPPER
> 4 red snapper fillets (4 oz each)
> ¼ cup fresh lime (or lemon or orange) juice
> 1 tbsp fresh lemon juice
> 1 tsp chili powder
> Red pepper flakes (few) or dash tabasco sauce
> 1 plum tomato coarsely chopped (fresh or canned)
> 4 green onions, sliced in ½ inch sections

Place red snapper in a shallow baking dish. Combine lime juice, lemon juice and chili powder in a measuring cup. Pour over snapper. Marinate 10 minutes, turning once or twice. Sprinkle onions, tomato and peppers over snapper. Cover. Bake at 350 for 30 minutes or just until snapper flakes in center. Let stand, covered, 4 minutes before serving.

WHITE FISH, SERVED HOT OR COLD

½ to 1 lb white fish

Steam the fish until cooked through. Flake the fish and add:

½ tsp salt

Freshly ground white peppercorns

2 tbsp lemon juice or tarragon vinegar

½ cup ketchup (organic unsweetened)

2 or more tbsp capers

1 tbsp fresh horseradish

Dash of celery salt and cayenne pepper

Stir, taste for seasoning, and serve, or chill if desired. Garnish with parsley.

VARIATIONS:

Use barbecue sauce (see recipe below) or chili sauce instead of ketchup.

Add 1 tbsp or more of any of the following: chopped onions, cheeped leeks, chopped chives or green onions.

Omit capers and season with 1-3 tsp minced fresh fennel, dill, marjoram, or thyme; or add ½ tsp anise, dill or celery seeds.

Instead of fish, use steamed shrimp, flaked crab, lobster, or clams.

WHITEFISH MEDITERRANEAN
>Whitefish
>1 large tomato, cut in chunks
>Onion
>Vegetable broth (save broth from cooked or steamed veggies)
>Lemon juice
>Garlic, minced
>Sea salt
>Freshly ground black pepper

Sauté onion in some vegetable broth and lemon juice. Add fish, garlic, tomatoes, salt, and pepper. Add tomatoes and cook for 2-3 minutes until cooked thoroughly.

Maintenance and Forever After Version: Sauté onion in a little butter. Add fish, tomatoes, spices, and ½ cup of half and half.

GRILLED MAHI MAHI
>Mahi Mahi
>Fresh lime juice
>Garlic, minces

Marinate fish in lime juice and garlic for about 5 minutes and them put it on the grill.

SHRIMP SCAMPI
>6 jumbo shrimp, frozen or thawed
>¾ to 1 cup tomatoes
>½ tsp onion powder
>½ tsp chopped garlic or garlic powder
>Juice from ½ lemon
>Fry the shrimp with the lemon juice. Add tomatoes and spices and cook until shrimp is cooked.
>Shrimp and Tomato

Shrimp
Fresh lemon juice
Garlic, chopped
Red pepper flakes
1 fresh tomato or 2 canned tomatoes

Cook the shrimp in a pan with a little water, lemon juice, garlic, pepper flakes, and tomato for 5 minutes.

SHRIMP WITH ASPARAGUS

Shrimp or fish
Asparagus
Garlic, minced
Fresh lemon juice
Spices of choice

Grill shrimp, or fish, with asparagus, garlic, lemon juice, and spices for 5 minutes.

GRILLED WHITE FISH OR SHRIMP

3 to 6 oz. Fresh white fish or shrimp
Key lime juice or fresh lemon or lime juice
Garlic, minced
Sea salt
Fresh ground black pepper

Marinate fish in lime juice, lots of garlic, salt, and pepper for 20 minutes. Marinate shrimp 5 minutes. Grill. Shrimp can grill in 2 minutes.

SEA BASS WITH GARLIC AND TOMATOES

Garlic
Tomatoes, diced
Sea salt
Fresh ground black pepper

> Clogged with yesterday's excess, the body drags the mind down with it.
>
> **Horace**

211

Brown both sides, then add the tomatoes and garlic.

Cook in frying pan until fish is cooked through.

Recipe Courtesy of Rhoda:

POACHED FISH
Unsweetened, organic tomato sauce and tomato paste
Green beans
Onion- at least ½ an onion–red onions are best
Garlic–3 or 4 cloves, sliced thin
Filleted white fish (sole, tilapia, etc.)
Salt, pepper, basil

In a large non-fat skillet, sauté onion and garlic until golden. Don't let the garlic burn.

Add 1 can of tomato sauce, about 4 tablespoons tomato paste.

Add a little water if too thick.

Add green beans (if using frozen, partially thaw first)

Add basil, salt and pepper.

Place fish filet pieces on top of mixture, and place lid on pan, cook only for about 6 to 8 minutes until fish is white inside.

Beef

ROAST BEEF AND COLE SLAW WRAP
3 to 6 oz. Lean sliced roast beef
Cabbage, finely shredded
Apple cider vinegar
Bragg's amino acids

Mustard, Dijon or brown
Garlic, minced
Celery salt
Fresh ground black pepper

Combine all except beef. Roll up the beef with the coleslaw inside and eat cold.

BUFFALO BURGERS

6 oz leanest buffalo
Tomato (counts as your fruit)
Red onion (optional)

Form into a patty and grill. Top with sliced tomato and red onion if mixing vegetables.

MEATLOAF

1 lb lean ground beef or buffalo
1 tsp freshly ground black pepper
2 cloves garlic, minced
1 or 2 tbsp onions, minced
¼ tsp mustard powder
2 tbsp tomato paste

Mix all ingredients in bowl. Form into loaf and put in baking pan or loaf pan. Bake at 350 degrees 30-45 minutes.

May add other seasonings to change taste.

SLOW ROASTED CHUCK ROAST

Chuck roast, best with bone in
1 cup dry red wine
2 cups chopped tomatoes (optional) (tomato used as a fruit)
3 tbsp garlic or garlic powder
1 bay leaf

2 tbsp herbs de provence, or 1 tbsp each rosemary and basil

2 sliced leeks or small sliced onion or 2 tablespoons onion powder

1 cup baby carrots

Salt and fresh ground black pepper to taste

Marinate Chuck Roast in red wine and herbs for 1-2 days in refrigerator. Place vegetables in bottom of crock pot and place meat on top. Pour over marinade and add water until liquid reaches to top of meat. Cook on low 8 or more hours.

FLANK STEAK WITH NECTARINES

1 ½ pound beef flank steak

4 nectarines, each cut in half

¼ cup red wine

¼ cup soy sauce

¼ cup chicken broth

½ tsp Stevia

½ tsp ground ginger

2 cloves garlic, minced

Make cuts about 1/2" apart and 1/8" deep in a diamond pattern on both sides of the beef. Place beef in a zip lock heavy duty plastic bag. Combine wine, soy sauce, chicken broth, honey, ginger and garlic in small bowl. Pour marinade over beef and seal bag. Place bag in glass baking dish to catch any leaks. Refrigerate for 4-24 hours.

When ready to grill, heat coals. Remove beef from marinade and reserve marinade. Grill beef 4-5" from medium heat for 12-14 minutes until medium doneness, brushing twice with marinade and turning once. Add nectarines to grill for last 5 minutes of grill time, turning once and brushing frequently with marinade. Discard leftover marinade. Cut beef across grain to serve. Serve with nectarines. 4 servings.

Pepper Steak with Apricots

> 1 cup no-fat chicken broth
> 1 cup orange juice
> ½ cup chopped apricots
> Pinch nutmeg
> Pinch salt
> 2 large New York strips steaks, each cut in half
> 4 tsp. Cracked black peppercorns
> 1 tbsp olive oil

In small saucepan, combine broth, juice and apricots. Cook until mixture is reduced and thickened, about 7-10 minutes. Add nutmeg and salt and set aside.

Meanwhile, press the pepper firmly into each side of the steaks. Brush grill rack with oil. Grill steaks over medium coals 8-10 minutes, turning once, until medium. Place on serving platter and pour warm apricot mixture over. Serve. Serves 4

A waist is a terrible thing to mind.

Tom Wilson

Chili

> 1 lb. ground Buffalo, or ground beef (very lean)
> 4 tsp tomato purée
> 2 16 oz large cans of Glen Muir fire roasted tomatoes or 2 large cans of Italian plum tomatoes, with or without basil
> 1 onion, peeled and finely chopped
> 2 cloves of garlic, crushed
> 1 tsp chili powder
> Cayenne pepper to taste
> ¼ tsp cumin

½ tsp oregano

½ tsp thyme

½ tsp basil

Sea salt to taste

Freshly ground black pepper to taste

Brown meat with onions and garlic and drain meat of fat. Add 2 cans of tomatoes, tomato paste, herbs and spices. Simmer for a few hours on low heat in large pan or place in crock pot and cook on low for 6-8 hours.

Chicken

TANGY CHICKEN

¼ Cup apple cider vinegar

3 tbsp mustard powder

3 cloves garlic, peeled and minced

1 lime, juiced

½ cup stevia

1 ½ tsp sea salt

Freshly ground black pepper to taste

6 chicken breasts or 12 tenders

In a large glass bowl, mix the cider vinegar, mustard, garlic, lime juice, lemon juice, Stevia, salt, and pepper. Marinate 8 hours overnight. Preheat an outdoor grill for high heat. Place chicken on the lightly oiled grill, (use spray oil) and cook 6 to 8 minutes per side.

SPICY STEVIA CHICKEN

2 tbsp stevia

2 tbsp fresh lemon juice

1 tbsp fresh orange juice

2 scallions, finely chopped or minced dried onions

1 tsp finely chopped fresh or dried thyme
1 tsp finely chopped fresh or dried sage
Freshly ground black pepper to taste
4 boneless, skinless, chicken breast halves (about
1 lb total)

In a large bowl combine stevia, lemon and orange juices, herbs, scallions, pepper. Put the chicken in the bowl and marinate for 1-2 hours. Fire up the barbecue and grill the chicken, turning constantly while basting with the marinade until the breasts are cooked. Or cook on indoor grill or in oven broiler.

Inspired by Adelle Davis

I am a huge fan of the nutritionist Adelle Davis. She inspired me to study nutrition. Her waffle recipe is the most delicious and healthiest in the world. Adelle's method of cooking meat at low temperatures makes even less expensive cuts of meat melt in your mouth.

Here are a few recipes adapted from Adelle's cook book "Let's Cook It Right."

SHISH KABOBS

Meat, chicken or shrimp
Cherry tomatoes
Onion
Asparagus
Herbs
Lemon juice

Cube chunks of beef, fish, or chicken. Use cherry tomatoes, chunks of onion, and chopped asparagus. Put on skewer. Season with herbs and lemon juice and grill 15 minutes.

BROILED CHICKEN

    Chicken breasts cut into 3 to 6 oz servings
    Apple cider vinegar
    Lemon juice
    Stevia
    Spices

Marinate chicken in vinegar, lemon juice, and Stevia. Add spices such as salt, pepper, curry, ginger, chili, and basil. Broil many of the servings together and bag them for later.

GRILLED CHICKEN BREAST

    Fresh rosemary
    Fresh garlic
    Coarse salt
    Pepper

Chop the rosemary, garlic and orange zest with the salt. Add the pepper. Rub mixture on raw chicken breast that has been seasoned with salt and pepper. Let it sit a while with the rub on it before cooking in a grill for 6 minutes.

STIR FRY

    Chicken or beef
    Green cabbage
    Onion
    Celery
    Broccoli
    Zucchini or yellow squash
    Bean sprouts
    Fat-Free Chicken Broth

Slice chicken and cabbage. Chop onion and celery small if mixing vegetables.

"Stir fry" with Coconut Vinegar or Chicken broth until veggies are tender

CHICKEN CHOW MEIN

Chopped cabbage
3 to 6 oz. Chicken Breast
1–2 tbsp Onion
Pinch of Ginger
Sea Salt
Pinch of Stevia

Chop cabbage, onions, and chicken. Place in a hot skillet and fry (keep it moving). Stir in spices. Cook until chicken is done, but not until the ingredients in the pan are dry.

CHICKEN ITALIANO

Chicken breast
1 tomato
Sea salt
Garlic
Pepper
Italian seasoning

Chop up the tomato and the chicken breast into bite size chunks. Place in a hot frying pan and stir fry with all the seasonings.

SAVORY CHICKEN

Chicken Breast
Celery
Onion
Sage
Poultry seasoning
Sea Salt
Freshly Ground Black pepper

Never eat more than you can lift.
Miss Piggy

219

Chop up chicken breast, celery, and onion, stir fry in heated skillet, adding seasoning to taste.

BAKED CHICKEN WITH APRICOTS

    ½ lb Fresh apricots, pitted and cut into quarters
    ⅓ cup chopped apricots
    ¼ cup minced onion
    ¼ cup orange juice
    1 tbsp Stevia
    ½ tsp Ground ginger
    1 tsp Dijon mustard
    2 lb split chicken breasts, bone in, skin on
    Salt and pepper to taste

Combine fresh apricots with dried apricots, onion, orange juice, honey, ginger and mustard in heavy saucepan. Bring to a boil, lower the heat and simmer for 10 minutes. Remove from heat and let cool.

Heat oven to 350 degrees. Season chicken with salt and pepper and place in a single layer, skin side down, in glass baking dish. Spread apricot mixture on top. Bake for 15 minutes, then turn chicken and baste. Increase temperature to 425 degrees and bake 15 minutes longer, until chicken is thoroughly cooked and juices run clear.

Source: Cooking With Fruit

RASPBERRY GLAZED CHICKEN

    ½ cup puréed raspberries, with ½ tsp Stevia mixed in
    1 tbsp Dijon mustard
    6 boneless, skinless chicken breast halves
    1-½ cup fresh raspberries

Prepare grill. Brush rack with vegetable oil. Mix raspberry jam and mustard. Place chicken on grill, cover and cook for 20-25 minutes, brushing frequently with the jam mixture and turning once, until juices run clear and center of chicken is no longer pink when thickest pieces are cut. Discard remaining jam mixture and serve chicken topped with raspberries.

PLUM BBQ CHICKEN KABOBS

> ½ cup puréed plum with 1 tbsp Stevia
> 2 tbsp Lemon juice
> 2 tbsp Soy sauce
> ¼ tsp Dried sage leaves
> 1 lb Boneless, skinless chicken breasts, cut into 1" pieces
> 1 cup seedless red grapes

In heavy duty zip lock plastic bag, combine preserves, lemon juice, soy sauce and sage leaves. Add chicken, seal bag, and turn to coat. Place in glass baking dish and refrigerate for 1-4 hours.

When ready to cook, heat grill. Drain chicken, reserving marinade. On each of five 12" metal skewers, alternately thread chicken pieces and grapes. Oil grill rack. Place kabobs on grill over medium heat 4-6" from coals. Cook 10 to 15 minutes, or until chicken is no longer pink, turning often and brushing frequently with reserved marinade. Discard any remaining marinade. Serves 5.

Recipes Courtesy of Deanna Noll:

CHICKEN BOWL

> 3.5 to 5 oz. Chicken breast, diced
> ½ to 1 cup water

Garlic, salt, pepper, paprika and other seasonings to taste

Serving of zucchini or other allowed vegetable serving, diced

Put chicken, water and seasonings in skillet. Cover and cook until done. Add zucchini and more water as necessary to keep a small amount of broth in pan. Cook until zucchini is tender and serve in a bowl with the broth.

This is also great as a "burger bowl" using very lean ground beef instead of chicken.

CHICKEN TACOS

Chicken breast, sliced in strips
Chicken broth or Bragg's amino acids or coconut
1½ tsp sea salt
1 tsp onion powder
1 tsp chili powder or ½ tsp. Red pepper flakes
1½ tsp cumin
½ tsp garlic powder
Chopped cilantro, if desired

For more spice, add a pinch of cayenne pepper.

Lettuce leaves, washed and dried, usually iceberg, but may use romaine leaves.

Saute Chicken in broth and add in the seasonings while it is cooking. Spoon in to lettuce leaves and wrap to eat. May add chopped onion or other veggies like chopped carrots to taste.

BLACKENED CHICKEN SEASONING

2 tsp paprika
1 tsp onion powder
1 tsp garlic powder

¼ tsp cayenne pepper

½ tsp white pepper

½ tsp black pepper

½ tsp sea salt

½ tsp thyme leaves, dried

½ tsp oregano leaves, dried

CHICKEN AND TOMATOES

Chicken breasts

Grape tomatoes

Stevia

Basil

1 tbsp apple cider vinegar

1 clove garlic, minced

Oregano

Lemon juice to taste

Sea salt

Freshly ground black pepper

Obesity is really widespread.

Joseph O. Kern II

Cook chicken on grill and put the 3 to 6 oz. portions into individual Ziploc bags and refrigerate. To prepare, dice a portion of chicken and put it in a bowl with a handful of sliced grape tomatoes. Mix it with Stevia, basil, apple cider vinegar, garlic, oregano, and lemon juice.

Beverages

GOOD MORNING SHAKE

> 6 large strawberries or ½ cup blueberries
> 1 rounded tbsp whey protein powder
> 8 oz spring or filtered water
> Stevia to taste
> 4 ice cubes

Mix together in blender until frothy. May substitute other berries for strawberries, or fresh peach.

REFRESHING SPARKLING SODA

> 8 oz Naturally carbonated Mineral water,
> Few Drops Flavored Stevia to taste (Sweet Leaf brand)
> Try Root Beer, Lemon, Orange
> Natural Lemonade
> Naturally carbonated Mineral water, 8 oz.
> Juice of ½ lemon
> Stevia to taste

NATURAL SPORTS DRINK

Same recipe as Lemonade. Add a pinch of sea salt to make sports drink.

HOT CHOCOLATE

> 6 oz. hot water
> Chocolate or chocolate mint stevia to taste

HERBAL COFFEE

Teecino Brand Flavored Herbal Coffees, brewed and sweetened with Stevia to taste. Teecino coffees available in Hazelnut, Vanilla Nut, Java

Desserts

RAW CINNAMON APPLESAUCE

    6 apples

    ½ tsp Stevia

    2-3 tablespoons fresh lemon juice

Mix stevia and lemon juice. Core and slice apples. Mix with stevia and purée in blender just until smooth. Sprinkle with cinnamon and serve.

May also cook apples in a little water until soft to make traditional applesauce.

STRAWBERRY SMOOTHIE

    Strawberries

    Ice

    Stevia

Add some fresh squeezed lemon juice and a little water for a delicious 'daiquiri'. Put it in a goblet to make yourself feel special.

APPLE PIE

    Apple

    ¼ tsp cinnamon

    Dash Stevia

Cut apple into slices (pie style). Remove the core and seeds but don't peel. Arrange in a serving size Pyrex or ceramic bowl. Sprinkle with cinnamon and Stevia. Bake in 375 degree oven for 20 minutes. Use the liquid English Toffee flavored Stevia or Pumpkin Pie spice for variety. Or coat it with lemon and sprinkle with allspice.

FRUIT COBBLER

Almost any fruit can be turned into a delicious dessert. The best choices would be seasonal, fresh fruit, organic if possible. Frozen fruit may be used in a pinch. Strawberries, blueberries, blackberries, apples, peaches, pears are all good choices.

For each serving allow one whole fruit or handful of berries.

Preheat oven to 375 degrees. In a baking dish slice the fruit. You may peel or not, as you wish.

For each serving or fruit use 1 tsp. of fresh lemon juice. Put lemon juice into a small bowl. Add Stevia. You may use lemon, vanilla or orange Stevia. Or you may use powdered. Try ½ dropper of liquid Stevia or 1 tbsp of powdered. (You may need to experiment with this, as I find that different brands have various degrees of sweetness.) Add ¼ tsp. Vanilla, if using plain or lemon Stevia. Add a ¼ tsp fresh ground Nutmeg and 1/2 tbsp Cinnamon.

Mix together and sprinkle over the fruit. Bake until fruit is cooked but still firm.

For Phase 3, add 1/2 tsp melted butter and 2 tbsp almond or hazelnut meal for each serving of fruit. You may grind your own nut meal from raw or roasted nuts. Or look for bags of ground nut meal in health food store or online. Mix nut meal in bowl with Stevia and flavorings and sprinkle over fruit. You may also sprinkle some coarsely ground nuts on top of the fruit for crunch. This makes a gluten and sugar free dessert that is yummy enough for company.

MOCK CHOCOLATE PUDDING (RHODA)

  ½ to ⅓ cup of unsweetened, well-chilled
  applesauce (only apples, no other ingredients)–
  1 teaspoon Hershey's unsweetened cocoa powder
  Sprinkle of cinnamon
  ½ packet Stevia

Stir very well, until all the cocoa is incorporated and the mixture is smooth

STRAWBERRY DESSERT (RHODA)

  Frozen strawberries
  Hershey's unsweetened cocoa
  Stevia (few drops)
  Vanilla extract (few drops)

Mix cocoa, stevia and vanilla extract until thick and smooth. Dip or roll frozen strawberries into the mixture and then refrigerate. The strawberries will thaw slightly, and the cocoa mixture will harden around the berries. Makes a great treat!

STRAWBERRY SORBET (DEANNA)

  Portion of strawberries
  1 tsp of lemon juice
  ¼ to ½ cup of water
  ½ packet of Truvia

Stem and freeze portion of strawberries.

In a blender, place frozen strawberries, lemon, water and Truvia. Purée.

Put mixture in container and freeze. The amount of time in freezer will determine consistency of sorbet – from slushy to frozen.

When I buy cookies I eat just four and throw the rest away. But first I spray them with Raid so I won't dig them out of the garbage later. Be careful, though, because that Raid really doesn't taste that bad.

Janette Barber

PHASE 3 RECIPE

CRUST-LESS HIGH PROTEIN QUICHE

¾ cup beef, chicken or seafood of choice
¾ cup vegetables of choice
½ cup cheese
4 eggs
1 to 1 ½ cups of cream, milk, unsweetened soy, or a combination.

Prepare the solid ingredients–sauté and season any raw meats and vegetables. About 1 to 1½ cups of these work well for one quiche–more if there is no or little cheese. About 1½ to 2 cups total solid ingredients for a 9" pie pan is about right.

Spread meats and vegetables into a deep-dish pie pan.

Spread shredded cheese on top of the other ingredients.

Make the custard, using either a bowl with whisk, or (my favorite) a blender. A standard quiche might use 4 eggs to 1 and 1/2 cups of liquid, and this amount works well for a deep-dish 9" pie pan. You can use cream, milk, unsweetened soy milk, or a combination. Include seasonings as desired. I usually use salt, pepper, an herb or two if not already in the pan, and perhaps some dried mustard powder.

Pour the custard over the solid ingredients, and put onto center rack of 375 F. oven for 30-45 minutes.

Success Stories

JUST WANTED TO LET YOU KNOW HOW HAPPY I HAVE BEEN with the results of the HCG diet. After several months of normal eating (yes, I have cut down on bread and sugar, and am eating more fruit) I have maintained a very stable weight with minor fluctuations of 2-3 pounds from my goal weight of 185. This is truly amazing as in the past, every diet I have attempted simply saw the pounds pile back on within weeks of getting back to "normal." J.C.

TODAY WAS DAY 40. I WENT FROM 137.8 TO 118.1 SO I'VE lost 19.7. I am wearing jeans I wore 20 years ago and I've actually lost so much weight that my nice pumps don't fit me anymore HA HA! I look great!

BTW, my 22 year old daughter has had a chronic weight problem for most of her life. She's shorter than I and, at her heaviest, weighed about 220 pounds. She just started maintenance today. She lost a total of 30 lbs and 50 odd inches! She's really winning on this diet and I can't tell you how thankful I am as her mom! M.N.

> If nature had intended our skeletons to be visible it would have put them on the outside of our bodies.
>
> Elmer Rice

I CHANGED MY DIET FOR THE BETTER DRAMATICALLY. I learned to control my eating habits better. I also lost 9 lbs and looked much better. I handled problem areas (my lower body) that I hadn't been able to handle otherwise. I definitely suggest people do it as it's an effective way to address not only weight, but health. A.R.

DR. DUNEV HAS BEEN MY HOMEOPATH FOR OVER A YEAR when she asked if I needed any help with any other body problems (as she had already helped my sinuses, digestion and neck problems). I grabbed my belly fat and said jokingly "yeah, get rid of this" and to my great surprise and delight, she did that and more. She introduced me to the Homeopathic HCG and this was in Nov. of '09 and I weighed 149.5 and by January 1st I had lost 20 lbs. I only planned on losing about 10 lbs but it was so easy and healthy, I just kept going and losing more and more. I even stopped for Christmas and did eat some goodies, and still lost weight. I keep my weight between 131 and 134 all the time. If I should put on some extra weight I do a short term version of the diet, which I LOVE TO DO, and the weight falls off of me. I tell everyone what a "forgiving diet" this is. It's easy, healthy and fun. Oh yeah, I had some great side benefits from the weight loss too. I stopped eating processed foods and wheat w/gluten and my arthritis in my hands healed. I swear to you it's all gone. AND I lost at least 4 inches in my waist and went from a size 12 to 6.

Thank you Dr. Anne Dunev for my great shape and healthy body. B.L.

FIRST OF ALL, I WANT TO SAY THAT I WAS QUITE SURPRISED at how easy this diet was. I first noticed that I was feeling the muscles in my legs and thighs. Then I noticed that my frame was smaller all around. The fat wasn't just coming off in one place. The whole shape of my body was getting smaller overall. I was very certain that it wasn't just water weight.

My face got smaller and I was able to see my bone structure. This occurred uniformly throughout my body.

I will say it is the most successful diet I have every tried and it is the ONLY diet that I have ever done for 26 days plus the maintenance. I never thought that it was possible for me. D.F.

I JUST WANTED TO SHARE MY SUCCESS ON DOING THE HCG drops. I have been doing the diet for 26 days and during this time I have felt huge physical and mental improvement and it has reduced my food cravings.

I have lost about 18 lbs total on this program (I actually changed my eating habit before I started and lost an additional 7 lbs prior by staying off sugar and carbs). I have clearly seen how the HCG program has had a positive effect on my body as I get less tired, and my period has become normal (whereas before it wasn't).

In the past I had done different types of diet programs, but I had never felt that I was going to be able to make it. On this program I felt it early on and saw the obvious success even when I had just started and only been on a couple days.

Thank you so much for whoever developed this product, this really works. M.C.

THE HCG DIET WAS VERY EASY. I THOUGHT WHEN I started I'd only be able to survive the 26 days, but I ended up just doing the 43 days with no problem. Also, I've actually NEVER done a diet so successfully. I lost 20 lbs total after YEARS of not being able to lost weight! I'm SO glad I did this. I also had the luck of toning up just from doing it.

My skin actually tightened! I'd recommend this diet hands down! F.L.

I'VE HAD HIGH BLOOD PRESSURE FOR YEARS. I'VE BEEN taking medication for it. Since being on the HCG diet, my blood pressure went down to normal and NEVER went back up. It's been 4 months now that I've been off medication and my blood pressure is still normal! D.E.

I LOST 23 POUNDS, I WENT FROM A SIZE 38 TO A 34 IN 3 weeks and am in better physical shape than I've ever been since I was a teenager and if someone told me this was going to happen this effectively I would have thought they were sincerely lying. But if you look at the picture of stand by the scale you would see a miracle. Thank you. J.R.

I LOST 22 POUNDS, AND ISSUE I WAS HAVING WITH HIGH blood pressure disappeared and my blood pressure stabilized in a normal range. I am able to fit in clothes that I haven't been able to wear in years. This definitely went above my expectancies of the diet. Thank you. C.Z.

I LOST 25 POUNDS, GOT RID OF FAT THAT I'VE NEVER BEEN able to get rid of and I feel great. Thank you. R.K.

I LOST 13 POUNDS AND ABOUT 2 DRESS SIZES. SINCE completing the diet have maintained about a 10-13 pound loss with little fluctuation beyond that. I have not been this size since high school. I also noticed my period since then has not been painful (no cramps) and lasted only 4 days, with the first day being heavy but light after that. It seemed like how it should be, normal (prior to this my period would got on for a week and I would experience cramps on the first day and sometimes on the second day).

I am happy with the diet and never felt like I was suffering through it. I even cheated once or twice and still did well on it. I was worried too about the maintenance part as I had to leave town the day I started it and was on the road for almost the entire 3 weeks on the maintenance program, but as I stated above I managed to stick within some realm of the rules for that part of the diet and I am still maintaining my weight as we speak. I have been promoting the heavily to others as the diet to do, it seems very healthy and I am happy. I play to do it again in the near future, to get down to my ideal weight (another 10 pounds or so).

We never repent of having eaten too little.

Thomas Jefferson

As a further success and proof of this, which got me started on it… my sister did this diet after years and years of trying everything else under the blue moon and sun, and it was the only thing I saw stably work for her and so far she has kept it off. This was a success for her and I know it can work for anyone if they can just tough it out the 3 weeks and do it. –V

I ended up losing a total of 22 pounds and 33 inches, going from a size 6/8 to a 1/2. I personally have put about 40 friends, family and acquaintances on this miraculous diet and we LOVE it! M.L.

ZOE LOST 60 POUNDS AND IS ALMOST WEARING A SIZE 12. For the first time since she was a little girl, she can actually enjoy shopping in a mall and going to trendy stores, rather than going to plus size stores! M.L.

I WAS ON HCG FOR 1 MONTH AND WENT FROM 160 TO 145 in 30 days. Early on, I did experience some hunger; after the first week it went away. I have maintained my weight by eating a high protein diet. I have excluded all processed foods. I do not eat any "white" flour nor do I drink diet soft drinks or use any sugar substitutes other than stevia. I am a widow and I don't really have any recipes as I cook for myself and keep it simple and healthy. I find if I do get hungry, I grab a boiled egg and a few melba toast whole grain crackers. This is the only diet I have had any long term success with. While on the diet, I did avoid any meals out but if I could not avoid it, I stuck with protein, no sauces and steamed veggies which most restaurants could accommodate. I highly recommend this diet and Dr. Dunev as she is very understanding and compassionate. C.M.

I FOUND OUT ABOUT HCG DIET THROUGH A FRIEND. Advertisements don't impress me. I don't know personally any of these people. With so much scam, you just can't be sure. But seeing the dramatic results on someone you know makes a statement. I found out more details as to the theory of the diet. For the first time in trying countless plans I knew this was different. I took a chance. I never looked back. It had the key points to close me. 1. Price was right. 2. Simple. 3. Results right away. There's a lot of programs out there. They may have 1 or 2. But all 3?— not that I have discovered in my 25–30 years of looking.

There is something to be said for gratification and confidence of getting the weight off in a healthy manner and keeping it off in relative short time span. You can't beat that. C.J.

AT THE AGE OF 58, I FOUND MYSELF ABOUT 40 POUNDS overweight and no real hope of getting rid of the weight, but I knew that I had to some how get if off or face things like High Blood Pressure, Stroke, Heart Attack or Type 2 Diabetes. I was not having a good time with all the weight and my knees started to hurt me. I did not want a life of taking medication for any of the above, if I could help it. But what to do? I tried to stop eating at night after 7:00 p.m. I cut back on carbs and sugar, but NOTHING.

Yes, I had done diets before, but the weight always crept back on and I was back to where I was again, especially after the age of 45. Nothing seem to help, until my friend told me about the HCG Diet.

So, I ordered the drops (Homeopathic) and read Dr. Simeons' book "Pounds and Inches."

I read it, then read it again to make sure that I really had the information. Then I started.

I did my first round and lost 25 pounds in 32 days and lost over 40 inches from neck down. I was blown away with the results. Did the maintenance program, which I did NOT gain anything, then back onto round 2. On round 2 I lost another 18 pounds in 30 days and lost about several more inches.

I have now been off the diet since May 25th 2010 and have maintained my weight. This was incredible. I eat a bit different, but I will do some starches and sugar, but not that much. I eat well, protein, veggies and fruit. I have not cut out all starches or sugar, but I don't crave it. I weigh myself everyday and I have not gained more than 1.5 pounds, and that normally comes off the next day. I do still drink a lot of water, but I live in Nevada and it's vital!

I can say one thing…THIS DIET WORKS. I feel great and my knees feel good again!! R.F.

THANKS SO MUCH FOR GREAT HOMEOPATHIC VERSION OF the HCG diet. To me, this is the way to do the diet; no actual hormones; increased calories allowed; and no "low-havingness" on food. This protocol made it easy to lose weight . . . and I "cheated" regularly! For one thing, I had my SuperFood/Standard Process Whey Protein every day (sometimes twice). You even told me how to adjust the diet so I could exercise more; this was appreciated.

I had a big win, losing about 25 pounds, and, more importantly, lots of inches! I went from a size 42 suit to a size 38; from a 34" waist to a 32/31"; I replaced virtually my entire wardrobe! It was a win to be able to once again wear some Coach belts that had been hanging in my closet for over 20 years. The HCG diet simply works; the weight melts off; at one point during my second time on the diet, I thought it might be coming off too fast, if you can believe that!

All one has to do is follow your instructions and they will have a nice win.

Thanks very much! M.G.

"I'VE BEEN TRYING TO LOSE WEIGHT FOR YEARS. I WASN'T a yo-yo dieter, since I had NO success, and nothing ever came off for me to put back ON again! My metabolism is very bad—I am hypothyroid and have been on thyroid medication for years. It does nothing except satisfy the ranges on a lab report. When I went on the HCG diet, I was very skeptical. But I began losing right away. This was such encouragement! I was not hungry. I was able to completely change my eating habits with literally no trouble (I was previously a carb addict.) I've lost 25 pounds and feel good. During the maintenance phase, I add some allowed foods and still the weight doesn't come back. That's because one of the remarkable things about this diet is that if done correctly, it re-sets your metabolism. This is a great success for me—going from doing every diet I could find and taking losses as I lost NOTHING—to this tremendous accomplishment! Thanks, Dr. Dunev for the support along the way. This works!" RM

I HAD A BIG WIN, LOSING ABOUT 25 POUNDS, AND, MORE importantly, lots of inches! I went from a size 42 suit to a size 38; from a 34" waist to a 32/31"; I replaced virtually my entire wardrobe! It was a win to be able to once again wear some Coach belts that had been hanging in my closet for over 20 years. The HCG diet simply works; the weight melts off; at one point during my second time on the diet, I thought it might be coming off too fast, if you can believe that!

I'm allergic to food. Every time I eat it breaks out into fat.

Jennifer Greene Duncan

All one has to do is follow your instructions and they will have a nice win.

Thanks very much! M.G.

I AM DOING WELL—I HAVE LOST ABOUT LBS WHICH I AM really happy about. I am feeling very good and owe it all to you! E.K.M.

I HAVE LOST 35 POUNDS AND 4 DRESS SIZES, IN A MATTER of months on the HCG diet. This has been the most successful diet I have ever done.

I have failed at every diet I've attempted. I've never lost more than 10 pounds at a time and always gained it back. Until I did the HCG diet. This diet gives you exact guidelines to follow, and if followed, the weight loss is amazing!

This was surprisingly an easy diet to follow. The hunger and cravings went away and the weight loss was so steady that it kept me determined! Which has always been my problem in the past. It still to this day, I haven't gained back a single pound lost! I would recommend this diet to everyone! If I can have this kind of success I think everyone can! S.L.

I HAVE SEEN REALLY GREAT RESULTS FROM THE HCG drops and new lifestyle. I think my eating habits are what really helping things out for me. I've seen almost a 20 pound weight loss! F.N.

THIS IS THE ONLY DIET I HAVE EVER DONE THAT I'VE actually been able to stick to. On this diet I was having daily wins that kept me motivated to stick to it. I lost a lot of weight and felt healthy and energetic while doing it. My skin even cleared up! I would recommend this diet to anyone who wants to lose weight in the exact right areas and feel healthy while doing so. C.M.

JUST WANT TO SHARE MY WINS ON TAKING HCG DROPS. I have been doing the 26-day program on this diet and all the while I feel I am physically and mentally improving. It also reduces my cravings.

I lost about 18 pounds total. I get less tired and my period has been much more normal.

In the past I had done a different type of diet program, but I never had the certainty that I would be able to make it. But this program had obvious success after just the first couple of days, and I knew this program was going to work-and it did!

I am happy I had a chance to do this program. Thank you so much for developing this product-it really works. M.C.

Just a note to say "Hello!" and thank you for your help. I was very successful with the diet and lost 19 lbs in 4 weeks. I am very happy with the results and am on maintenance now. It is interesting to see the difference in the body by eating this way. It seems much more natural and suitable to the body's processes. My menopausal symptoms have also diminished to almost nothing in the course of this. I am hoping that remains stable now that I'm off the drops. Thanks again! R.K.

GLOSSARY

ADRENALIN – Hormone produced by the inner part of the Adrenals. Among many other functions, adrenalin is concerned with blood pressure, emotional stress, fear and cold.

ADRENALS – Endocrine glands. Small bodies situated atop the kidneys and hence also known as suprarenal glands. The adrenals have an outer rind or cortex which produces vitally important hormones, among which are Cortisone similar substances. The cortex is the inner part of the adrenals, the medulla, secretes adrenalin and is chiefly controlled by the autonomous nervous system.

AUTONOMOUS NERVOUS SYSTEM – That part of the nervous system that acts as a control in maintaining homeostasis (stable, constant condition) in the body. These activities are generally performed without conscious control or sensation. The ANS affects heart rate, digestion, respiration rate, salivation, perspiration, diameter of the pupils, urination, and sexual arousal. Whereas most of its actions are involuntary, some, such as breathing, work in tandem with the conscious mind.

ARTERIOSCLEROSIS – Hardening of the arterial wall through the calcification of abnormal deposits of a fat-like substance known as cholesterol.

ASSIMILATE – Absorbed digested food from the intestines.

You know it's time to diet when you push away from the table and the table moves.

Quoted in *The Cockle Bur*

CALORIE – The physicist's calorie is the amount of heat required to raise the temperature of 1 cc. of water by 1 degree Centigrade. The dieticians's Calorie (always written with a capital C) is 1000 times greater. Thus when we speak of a 500 Calorie diet this means that the body is being supplied with as much fuel as would be required to raise the temperature of 500 liters of water by 1 degree Centigrade of 50 liters by 10 degrees. This is quire insufficient to cover the heat and energy requirements of an adult body. In the HCG method the deficit is made up from the abnormal fat deposits, of which 1 lb furnishes the body with more that 2000 Calories. As this is roughly the amount lost every day, a patient under HCG is never short of fuel.

CEREBRAL – Of the brain. Cerebral vascular disease is a disorder concerning the blood vessels of the brain, such as cerebral thrombosis or hemorrhage, known as apoplexy or stroke.

CHOLESTEROL – A fat-like substance contained in almost every cell of the body. In certain forms it can deposit along the inner lining of the arteries. No clear and definite relationship between fat intake and cholesterol-level in the blood has yet been established.

CHORIONIC – Of the chorion, which is part of the placenta or after-birth. The term is justly applied to HCG, as this hormone is exclusively produced in the placenta.

CONGENITAL – Any condition that exists before or at the time of birth.

CORTISONE – A synthetic substance which acts like an adrenal hormone. It is today used in the treatment of a large number of illnesses, and several chemical variants have been produced from it.

Diuretic – Any substance that increases the flow of urine.

Edema – An abnormal accumulation of water in the tissues.

Endocrine–Of or relating to the endocrine system.

Endocrine System – A system of glands in the body which each secretes vital hormones. These hormones are then carried through the blood to different parts of the body to regulate such things as mood, growth and development, tissue function and metabolism.

Gland–An organ in a body that creates a substance for release, such as hormones or breast milk, often into the bloodstream (endocrine gland) or into cavities inside the body or its outer surface.

Gonadotrophin – usually means hormones directed towards the testes or ovaries. However HCG acts, not on the reproductive organs, but on the hypothalamus gland, according to Dr. Simeons

HCG – An abbreviation of Human Chorionic Gonadotrophin.

Hormones – A kind of chemical released by certain parts of the body, which causes other parts of the body to react in response to this chemical.

Metabolism – The body's chemical turnover at complete rest and when fasting. The basal metabolic rate is expressed as the amount of oxygen used up in a given time. The basal metabolic rate (BMR) is controlled by the thyroid gland.

Migraine – A severe half-sided headache often associated with nausea and vomiting and sensitivity to light and sound.

Pituitary – Of or relating to the Pituitary Gland.

Pituitary Gland–A gland located at the base of the brain, which excretes hormones to control and regulate the other glands, and for this reason it is considered to be the "master gland".

Protein – from the Greek *protos* meaning "primary". It is the structural component of the body, such as muscle and collagen or connective tissue as well as enzymes. Every cell in the body has protein. The building blocks of protein are amino acids and there are 8 "essential" amino acids that human bodies cannot make and must derive from food sources.

Syndrome – A group of symptoms that are characteristic of a particular disorder. "Metabolic Syndrome" includes high cholesterol, high blood pressure, Diabetes, and obesity. The Fat Fix Diet plan has been shown to improve the symptoms of Metabolic Syndrome.

Bibliography

1. *Double Helix Water*, David L. Gann and Shui-yin Lo, D and Y Publishing, 2009

2. *Good Calories, Bad Calories*, Gary Taubes, Anchor Books, 2007

3. *Folk Medicine*, D.C. Jarvis, M.D., Ballantine Books, 1982

4. *The Metabolic Typing Diet*, William Wolcott and Trish Fahey, Random House, Inc. 2000

5. *Let's Get Well*, Adelle Davis, Harcourt, Brace, Jovanovich, 1965

6. *Good Foods, Bad Foods*, Judith A. DeCava, CNC, CCWFN, LNC, International Foundation for Nutrition and Health, 2009

7. *Let's Eat Right to Keep Fit*, Adelle Davis, Harcourt, Brace Jovanovich, 1954

8. *Nutrition and Physical Degeneration*, Weston A. Price, D.D.S., Price-Pottenger Nutrition Foundation, 1939

9. *Pottenger's Cats*, Francis M Pottenger, Jr. M.D., Price-Pottenger Nutrition Foundation, 1983

10. *Going Back to the Basics of Human Health*, International Foundation for Nutrition and Health, 1997

11. *Protein Power*, Mary Dan Eades, M.D. and Michael R. Eades, M.D., Bantam Books, 1996

12. *Excitotoxins: The Taste That Kills*, Russell L. Blaylock, M.D., Health Press, 1997

Distributors

If you would like to become a distributor and help others lose weight and become healthier, please contact me at this address: info@annedunev.com

California

Kay Curtis • Los Angeles, CA
Curtis Nutrition
www.CurtisNutrition.com
818-842-8921

Barbara Levine • Los Angeles, CA
www.noregretsdiet.com

Florida

Dr. Steve Lund • Clearwater, FL
727-492-0236

Jackie O'Meara • North Palm Beach, FL
Ocean Acupuncture of North Palm Beach
561-628-8701
www.oceanacu.com
oceanacu@comcast.net

Penny Jones • Clearwater, FL
727-412-4520
pennyjones1@mac.com

Georgia

Dr. Linda H. Katz • Fayetteville, GA
770-461-2225
Fayette Chiropractic Center

Amazon
Bio Source
$65 for
2 pack -
30 day supply
.5 mL
(10 drops)
3 X per day
15 min before meals

Kansas

Advanced Chiropractic Services
785-842-4181
Lawrence KS 66047
contact Melanie Wertin
Email melwertin@aol.com

Nevada

Ralynn Finn • Las Vegas, NV
702-292-9632
rmfinn@cox.net

Christine Juss • Las Vegas, NV
christinejuss@yahoo.com

Texas

Dr. James Franklin, DC • San Antonio, TX
210-341-5454

Dr. O C Pena, DC • San Antonio, TX
210-684-8575

Dr. Rene Ramon, DC • San Antonio, TX
210-657-6744

Penny Robinson • Corpus Christi, Austin or San Antonio, TX
361-236-3569
CalicoPenny@gmail.com

Taiwan

Yuen Li • Taichung
04-24368792 04-24360215
Fax 04-214366018
yinyun0410@yahoo.com.tw

Intolerances
Dairy 49

Plateau
* 49

Maint.
51-53

Suppl
53, 84

Prayer!
P 83 ?

Wt Gain
- Protein Soy
P 56

Debug
P 73

* Apple Day
132

P86 Candida + Probiotics

P84 Constipation

P91 Acid Reflux
P94

Liver / Gall Bladder Detox P64 - Dr Christophers

Standard Process.com - cleanses /detox Suppl.

CPSIA information can be obtained at www.ICGtesting.com
Printed in the USA
BVOW062041080912

299928BV00003B/2/P

9 780578 078472